All about nutrition for pregnant and breastfeeding women.

This material was developed by a certified nutritionist with input from dietitians, pediatricians, and breastfeeding specialists.

is presented as is, and while the author and publisher have made every effort to ensure accuracy, adequacy, completeness, legality, reliability, and usefulness, no warranty, express or implied, is given. We encourage you to accept all risks of using the information presented in this book. It is recommended that you consult a professional medical practitioner before embarking on any program or information in this book.

TABLE OF CONTENTS

FOREWORD

Dear mom-to-be,

I'm so excited to welcome you on this incredible journey! Motherhood, care, and love are waiting for you. Pregnancy and breastfeeding are times of amazing change, when our body and mind need special care and nourishment.

This book is your ultimate guide, your loyal companion in the world of nutrition during this incredible time. Get ready to discover the secrets of a healthy and balanced diet that will support you and your baby every step of this amazing journey!

We'll learn which nutrients are especially important during pregnancy and lactation, and which foods and meals to favor to keep your body strong and energized. We'll look at what elements affect your baby's health, and what nutritional principles will help you feel your best.

This book is so much more than just a reference book! It's a warm mentor who will be by your side every step of the way, sharing the joy of discovery and helping you overcome challenges. Being a mom is an amazing adventure, and together we can make it even more inspiring and unforgettable!

Let this book be your trusted guide in the world of caring for yourself and your baby. Let's create a healthy future together - for you, for your baby, and for your whole family.

With love and respect,
Valerie Spark

CHAPTER 1: THE BASICS OF HEALTHY EATING FOR PREGNANT WOMEN. THE IMPORTANCE OF A BALANCED NUTRITION DURING PREGNANCY. MYTHS ABOUT PREGNANCY DIET: WHAT TO AVOID.

A nutritious diet is one that includes a variety of

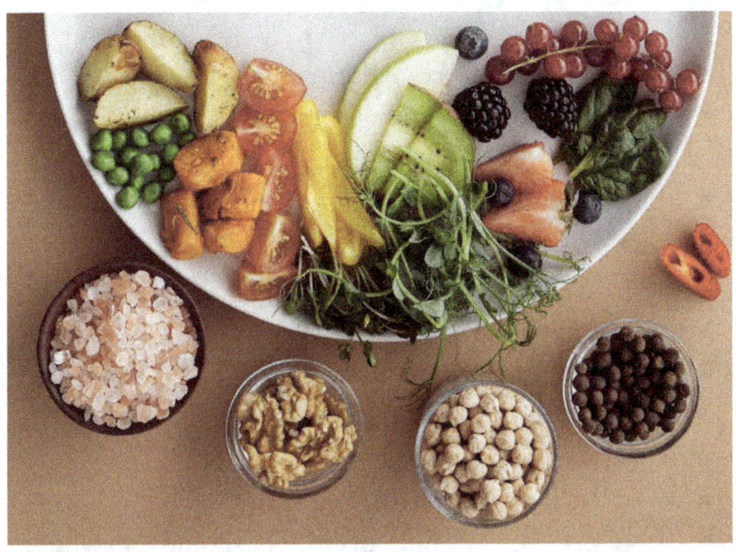

healthy foods from each food group. **In the first trimester**, you don't need to eat too many portions. **In the second trimester**, you need an extra 340 calories a day, and **in the third trimester**, you need about 450 extra calories a day. If a woman is carrying twins, she should get about 600 extra calories per day, and if she is carrying triplets, it is 900 extra calories per day.

Energy needs also vary depending on your pre-pregnancy body mass index, age, and level of physical activity.

Typical calorie requirements during pregnancy **range from 2200 to 2900 kcal/day** in the second and third trimester for individuals with a normal pre-pregnancy BMI.

You can calculate the calories you need using an online calculator. To do this, type "Pregnancy Calorie Calculator" or "Pregnancy Weight Gain Calculator" or "Calorie Calculator for Breastfeeding Moms" into the Internet search bar of your browser.

Must-have foods:
- **Vegetables of all kinds:** dark green, red, orange; beans, peas and lentils; starchy vegetables; and any other vegetables.
- **Fruits**, especially whole fruits.
- **Cereals**, and half of which should be whole grains.
- **Dairy products**, including low-fat or semi-skim milk, yogurt and cheese, as well as lactose-free and soy-fortified versions and yogurt as alternatives.

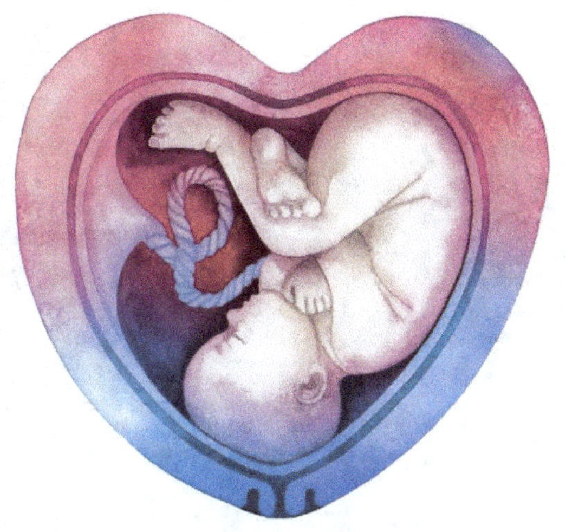

•   **Protein-rich foods**, including lean meat, poultry and eggs; seafood; beans and lentils; and nuts, seeds and soybeans.

•   **Oils**, including vegetable oils and oils in foods, such as seafood and nuts (but not tropical oils, which are high in saturated fatty acids).

There are foods that are recommended to be avoided during pregnancy.

Changes in the immune system of pregnant women increase the risk of foodborne illnesses for women and their unborn children. Some diseases of foodborne illnesses, such as Listeria and Toxoplasma gondii, can infect the fetus even if the mother does not feel sick.

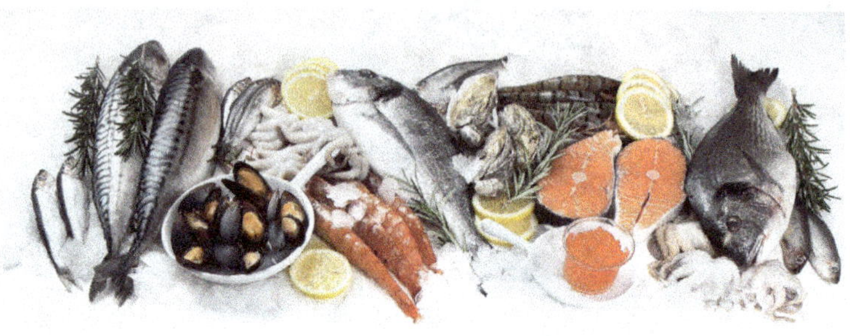

Seafood:

Fish is a source of high quality protein, minerals and vitamins that are beneficial for overall health. However, it is important to choose fish that is safe to consume and healthy.

Eating raw fish is a risk: raw fish or products made from raw fish are more often contain parasites or bacteria than foods made from cooked fish. Do not eat raw or undercooked fish or shellfish.

Cook seafood thoroughly: all seafood dishes should be cooked **at a temperature of 145° F** (64°C). Raw seafood may contain parasites or bacteria, including Listeria, which can cause illness of pregnant women and potentially harm their babies.

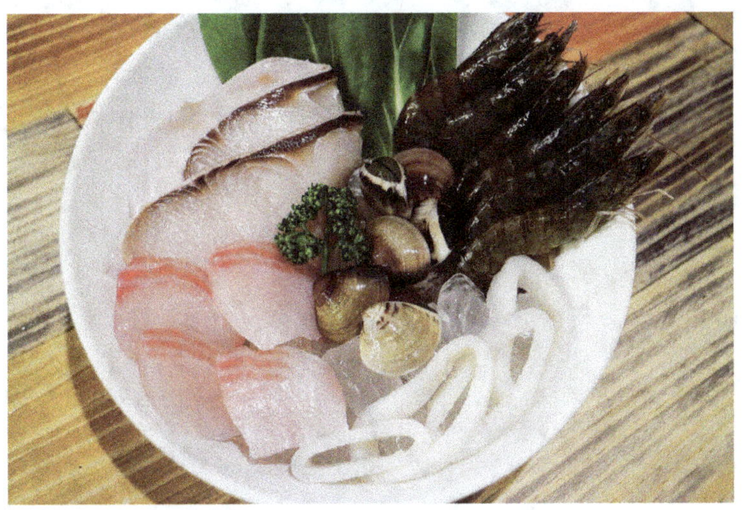

That means you should avoid foods like:

- Sushi
- Sashimi
- Raw oysters
- Raw shellfish
- Raw scallops
- and Ceviche

Be careful with smoked seafood:
Refrigerated smoked seafood poses a real threat. Do not eat refrigerated smoked seafood unless it is not in a cooked dish, such as a casserole, that reaches an internal temperature of 165°F (74°C) to kill harmful germs.

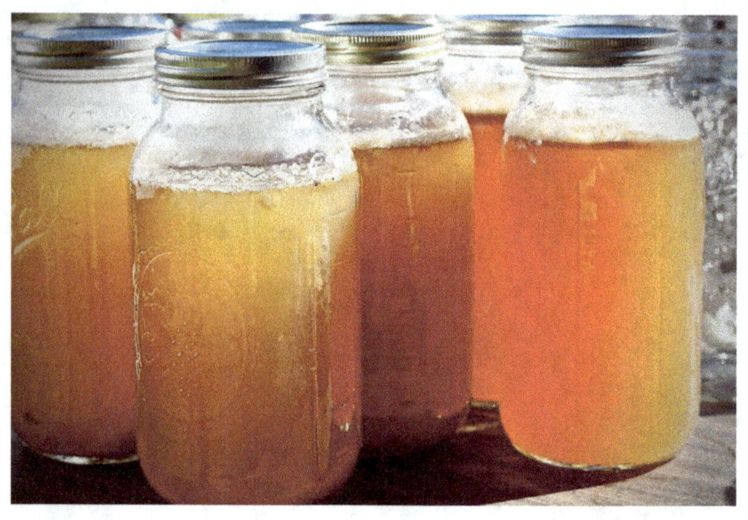

Do not drink unpasteurized juice or cider.
Unpasteurized juice, even freshly squeezed juice, and cider can cause foodborne illness. These beverages have been linked to outbreaks of E. coli and other harmful germs. To prevent infection, choose a pasteurized version or bring unpasteurized juice or cider to a boil and simmer for at least 1 minute before drinking.

Avoid raw milk, soft cheeses and other raw milk products.
Raw milk is the milk of any animal that has not been pasteurized to kill harmful bacteria. Raw milk, which is also called unpasteurized milk, can contain bacteria such as campylobacter, E. coli Listeria, Salmonella, or

even the bacteria that cause tuberculosis. To avoid foodborne illness, consume only pasteurized milk and dairy products, including cheese.

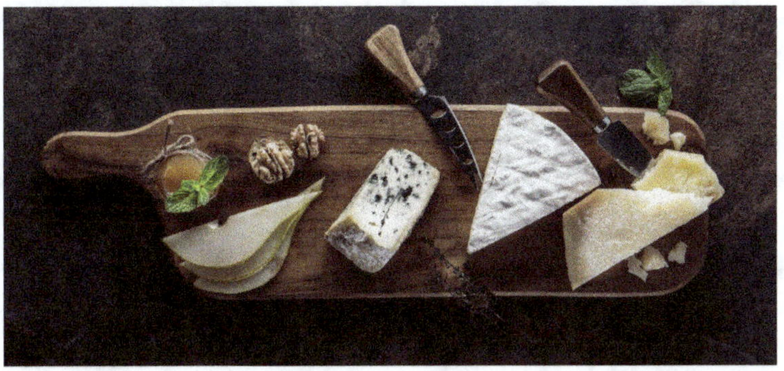

Avoid soft cheeses such as brie, feta, camembert, fresco, roquefort, unless they are made from pasteurized milk. The label should state that it is "made from pasteurized milk". To avoid foodborne illnesses, consume only pasteurized milk and dairy products, including hard cheese such as cheddar or Swiss.

Cook eggs thoroughly.
Undercooked eggs can contain salmonella, which can cause intestinal infections, which can be severe. If you are preparing a casserole or other dish containing eggs, make sure that the dish is cooked at a minimum of 165°F (71°C). This is important.

And, do not eat foods that may contain raw eggs, for example: homemade salad dressing Caesar, tiramisu, eggs Benedict, and homemade ice cream.

Avoid pre-packaged salads made from meat or seafood (e.g., chicken or tuna salads), which may also contain Listeria. Avoid raw sprouts such as alfalfa, clover, and radish, which may contain E. coli or Salmonella. Sprouts should be cooked thoroughly.

Avoid undercooked meat and poultry.

All meat and poultry should be thoroughly cooked to the minimum cooking temperature.

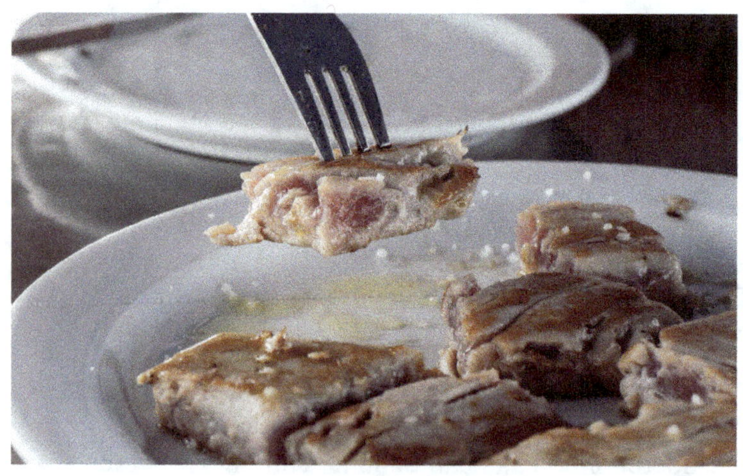

It is important to maintain the minimum recommended internal temperature, as meat and poultry may contain Escherichia coli, Salmonella, Campylobacter or Toxoplasma gondii.

Preventive measures to reduce the risk Toxoplasma infection through meat consumption:
- Cook meat to the minimum safe internal temperature.
- Freeze meat for several days at a sub-zero temperature of -0,4° F (-18 °C) before cooking to significantly reduce the likelihood of infection.
- After contact with raw meat, poultry, seafood, or unwashed fruits or vegetables, wash cutting boards, utensils, and equipment with hot water and detergent.
- Hand hygiene.

Avoid raw dough.
Raw dough or batter can cause a pregnant woman's illness, because the flour has not been processed to kill germs such as E. coli, and raw eggs are known to contain salmonella.
Make sure that the dough is is well baked or cooked.

Food in a restaurant: make sure that the food is thoroughly cooked, especially meat, poultry, fish, and eggs. When a hot dish is served, make sure it is hot and well cooked through.
Statistics show that pregnant women are 10 times more likely to get listeria than other people. This

infection can also cause miscarriages, stillbirths, premature births, serious illnesses, and even death in newborns.

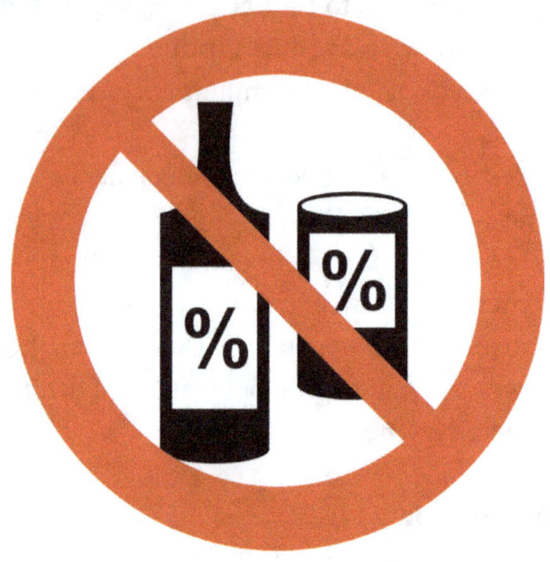

Alcohol:

Alcohol passes from the mother's bloodstream to the baby through the umbilical cord, just like everything else. Drinking alcohol during pregnancy can cause miscarriage, stillbirth, and a host of lifelong physical, behavioral, and intellectual disabilities. These disabilities are known as fetal alcohol spectrum disorders.

CHAPTER 2: THE IMPACT OF UNHEALTHY EATING ON MATERNAL AND CHILD HEALTH. CREATING A HEALTHY DIET FOR PREGNANT WOMEN. THE ROLE OF PROTEINS, FATS, CARBOHYDRATES, VITAMINS, AND MINERALS IN A PREGNANT WOMAN'S DIET.

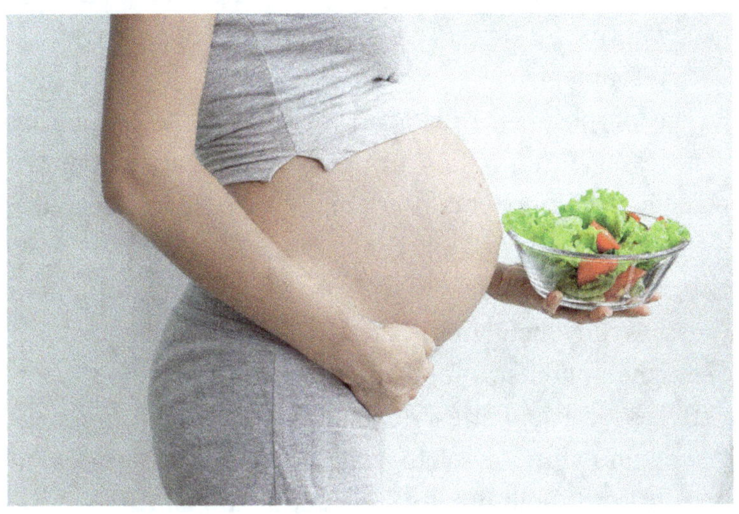

A healthy diet during pregnancy promotes fetal growth and development and is associated with a lower risk of pregnancy complications, while an unhealthy diet, malnutrition, and overnutrition are associated with adverse pregnancy outcomes. Adequate maternal intake of macronutrients and micronutrients contributes to normal embryonic and fetal development, while malnutrition and overnutrition (e.g., obesity) may be associated with adverse outcomes.

Such as: pregnancy and childhood, including miscarriage, certain congenital anomalies, hypertensive disorders of pregnancy, gestational diabetes, preterm birth, small for gestational age newborns, and suboptimal neurocognitive development.

The purpose of a dietary assessment is to obtain the necessary information from the current diet to identify dietary components that may increase or decrease health risks.

In addition to dietary assessment, it is important to assess key behavioral factors that are relevant to a pregnant woman's food choices.

Behavioral and lifestyle factors influence a pregnant woman's ability to change her diet and can be assessed by asking about previous dietary attempts.

Pregnant women should be asked about their dietary environment, which includes:

- Work and other time constraints, including weekends.

- Access, skills and financial capacity to purchase healthy foods.
- Time of intake - does the expectant mother not eat for hours and then increase her intake in the evening?
- Age and number of children living with the pregnant woman.
- Support from family members, including those who cook and buy food, because families are different and it is not always the woman who prepares meals. Sometimes it's the husband who cooks, and sometimes it's the mother-in-law, for example.
- Cultural and religious practices.
- Sleep, fatigue, stress, and illness.

In addition to assessing the diet, you need to take a medical history, possible illnesses and look at tests, if any. It is advisable not to eat three times a day, but 5-6 times a day in small portions. This is especially important in the second half of pregnancy. Macronutrients include proteins, carbohydrates, fiber and fats.

Proteins are high-molecular composed of amino acid residues linked in a specific sequence by peptide bonds. Proteins are essential substances without which life, growth and development of the body are impossible. Therefore, they cannot be absent from our diet, their presence **is important and necessary**.

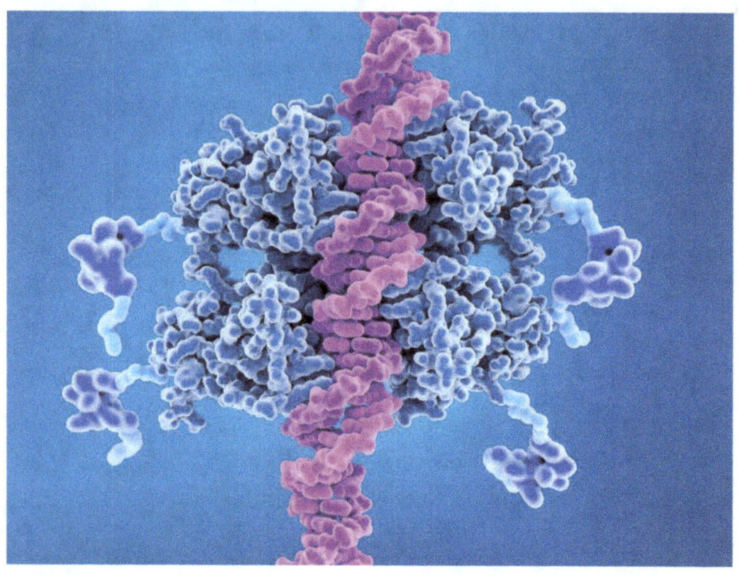

Protein is the main material for building cells. The full intrauterine development of a small human being requires the formation of billions of cells. **They are mainly used to build the cells of the tissues and organs of the unborn child, including the brain.** Protein also contributes to the growth of breast and uterine tissue during pregnancy and plays an important role in increasing blood supply. A baby uses about 35oz (1000 grams) of protein, with most of this need occurring in the last six months.

The recommended dietary allowance for protein during the second and third trimesters of pregnancy is 2.5oz (71 g)(approximately 0,04oz/1.1 g/kg/day).

Increasing protein intake should be proportional to total calories, as the percentage of calories from protein remains between 10 and 35 percent of total calories for both pregnant and nonpregnant individuals. Some experts recommend keeping protein intake below 25 percent of calories.

Healthy sources of protein include lean meats, poultry and eggs, seafood, beans, peas, lentils, nuts, seeds, and soy products.

Highly processed and fatty meats are not recommended.

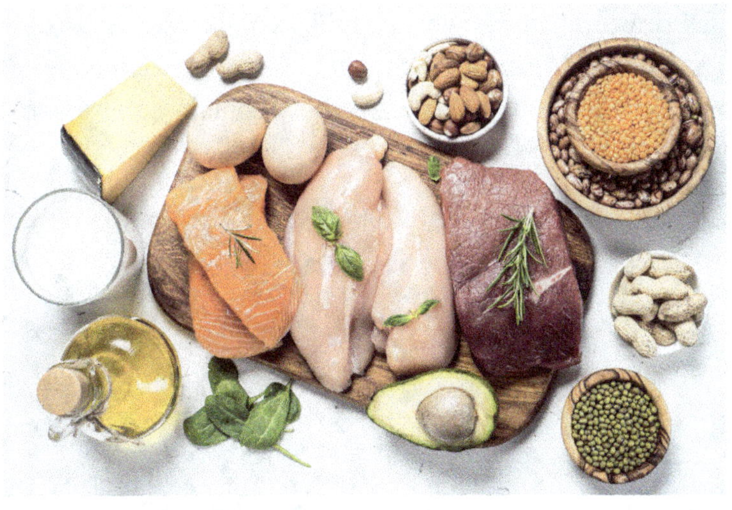

Meat is the most common source of protein.

Consuming meat helps to deliver proteins to the body quite efficiently because the components in meat are more similar to those found in our bodies. In other words, the body is able to use the building blocks of meat to build and maintain your body, as well as your baby's body.

Although meat is very healthy, it can cause its own complications. Therefore, it should be thoroughly washed before cooking. When cooking, make sure that the meat is well cooked. Meat should also be consumed in small quantities, as excessive consumption can lead to health problems. For example, eating liver, which is considered offal, can lead to birth defects and liver toxicity.

During pregnancy, you should avoid consuming too much fatty fish, such as trout, salmon, herring, and mackerel. This is because they contain toxins and pollutants.

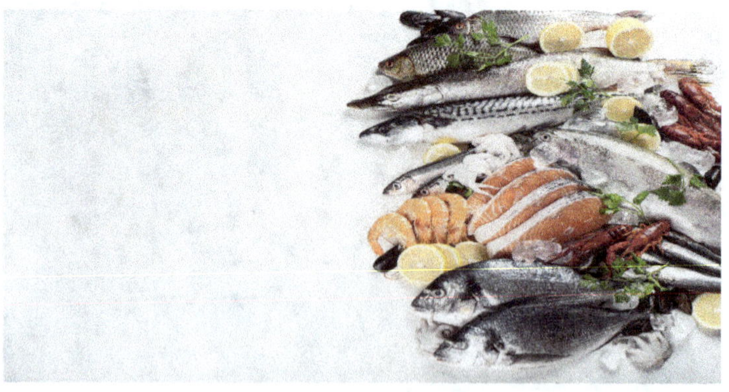

Legumes:

- Split peas;
- Red and white beans;
- Black beans;
- haricot beans;
- black-eyed peas;
- chickpeas (garbanzo beans).

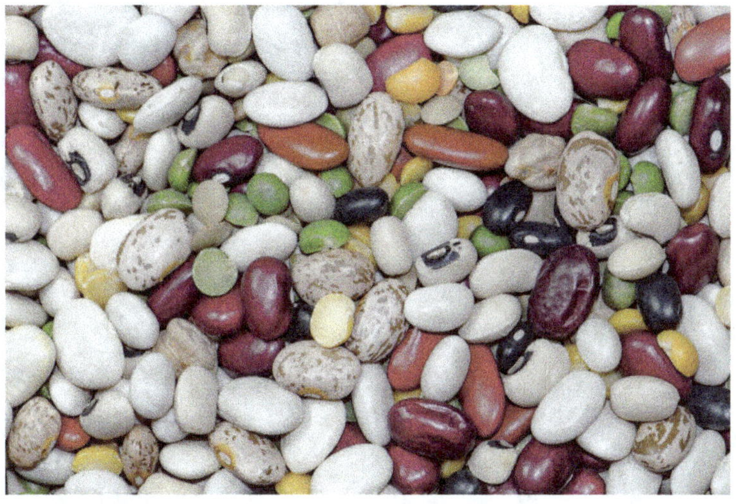

Dairy products such as cheese, milk, and yogurt are rich in calcium and very healthy. Consider choosing low-fat varieties, such as reduced-fat cheese, skim or semi-skim milk, or low-fat yogurt.

Cheese is a good source of protein, but soft cheeses should be avoided during pregnancy.

This is because it can contain listeria, harmful bacteria associated with the dangerous infection listeriosis.

Grains:
Most grains contain small amounts of protein. For example, one serving of quinoa contains up to 0.28oz (8 grams) of protein.

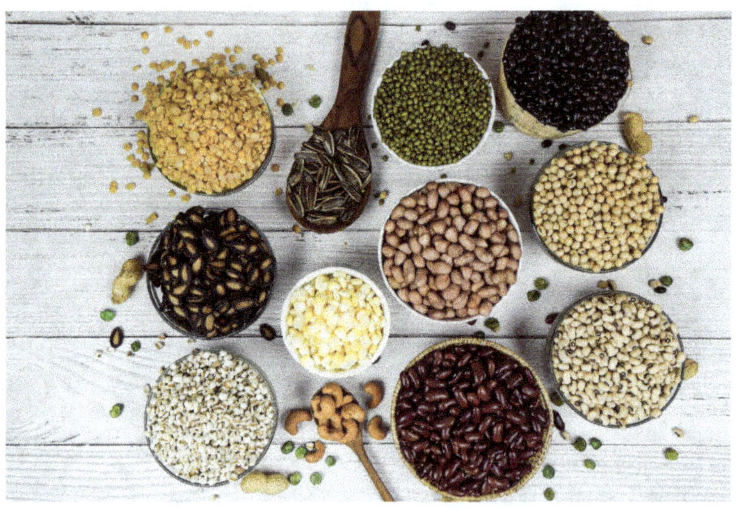

Carbohydrates are a source of energy and play an important role in many of the body's tissues. They are found in almost all foods except meat.
Sugar is also a pure carbohydrate, and neither the mother nor the fetus needs excessive amounts of it.

Therefore, by following a diet based on foods with a low glycemic index, which are foods that, when digested, provide a long-lasting feeling of satiety and prevent excessive blood sugar spikes, you can keep your blood sugar at a stable level, reduce the risk of developing gestational diabetes and other possible complications during pregnancy.

Foods containing starch are digested slowly, which means that energy is supplied to the baby's body slowly but constantly. **Highly processed carbohydrates should be minimized to help control weight gain** and avoid high blood glucose levels after meals, especially among those with diabetes or at high risk of developing it. **These include, for example, foods such as soda, mass-produced baked goods, candy, and sugar cereals.**

For pregnant women, carbohydrate needs increase to 6.2oz (175g) per day.

Dietary associations recommend 45 to 65 percent of calories to come from carbohydrates, as the increase in carbohydrate intake is proportional to the increase in calorie requirements during pregnancy.

Fiber-rich foods quickly fill you up and relieve hunger, and they also normalize the functioning of the gastrointestinal tract, slow the absorption of glucose, and are generally very important for the body. **Fiber is**

readily available and can be found in grains, legumes, fruits, vegetables, and nuts.

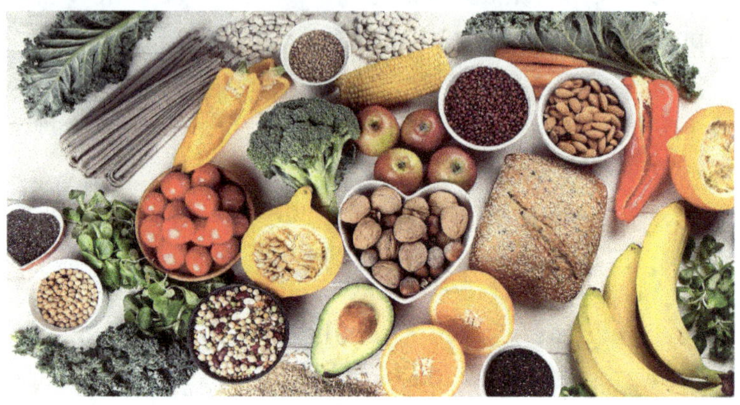

Fats in the diet of a pregnant woman should be of high quality only. From animal fats it is useful to use dairy fats - cream, sour cream, butter or ghee, and from vegetable fats - sunflower, corn, olive and soybean oil. Fats should be consumed in their natural form so that they do not lose their valuable properties.

To prevent fats from losing their valuable properties, they should be consumed in their natural form.
You can eat a salad with vegetable oil or a sandwich with butter every day, but it is advisable to eat hidden fats (sausages, meat sauces or muffins) in limited quantities.

And in the last trimester of pregnancy, a woman generally needs more fat than in the first two.
Long-chain polyunsaturated fatty acids are docosahexaenoic acid and eicosapentaenoic acid, also known as **omega-3**, which are mainly found in fish and seafood.

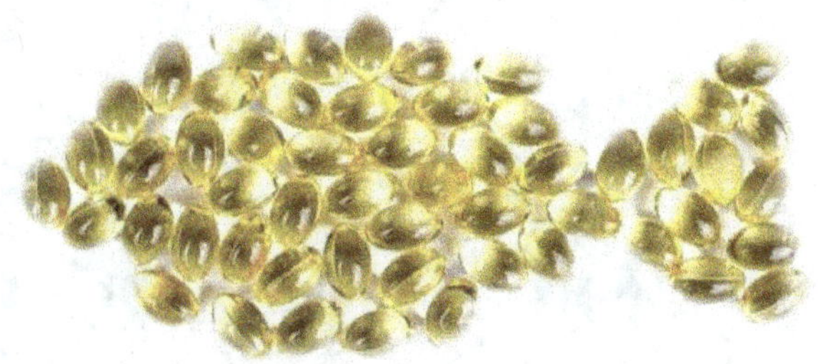

Docosahexaenoic acid is essential for normal development of the fetal brain and retina, and **seafood consumption during pregnancy is also associated with favorable cognitive development in the child.** Polyunsaturated fatty acids have anti-inflammatory properties.

Sources of omega are flaxseed (ground) or broccoli, cantaloupe, melon, beans, spinach, cauliflower, walnuts, and fish.

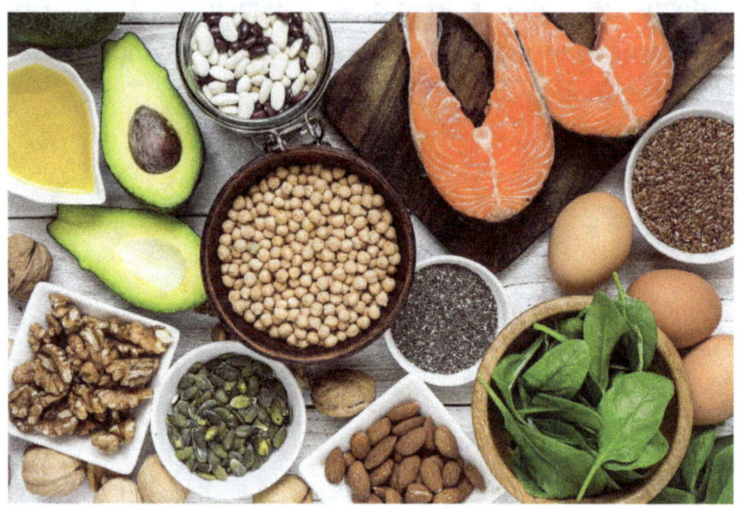

Dietary recommendations for pregnant women are to consume 8 to 12 oz (227-340 g) of seafood per week. The number of weekly servings of fish needed to achieve the target intake of polyunsaturated fatty acids is 200 to 300 mg/day.

Micronutrients

Iron is necessary for the development of the fetal brain and placenta, as well as for increasing the mother's red blood cell mass. Recommended intake:

The CDC recommends an iron intake of 27 mg/day during pregnancy, and the WHO recommends daily oral iron supplements containing 30 to 60 mg of elemental iron.

There are two dietary forms of iron: heme and nonheme.
The most bioavailable form is heme iron, which is found in meat, poultry, and fish. Non-heme iron, which makes up 60 percent of the iron in animal products, is less bioavailable. Absorption of non-heme iron is enhanced by consumption of vitamin C-rich foods or muscle tissue (such as meat, poultry, and seafood) and inhibited by consumption of dairy products and beverages such as coffee, tea, and cocoa.

Examples of daily sources of iron include
2-3 servings of green leafy vegetables (1 serving = about 1 cup)
- Beets
- Spinach
- Lettuce leaves
- Collard greens.

243 servings of whole grains
(1 serving = about ½ cup or one slice)
- Bread

- Corn Flour
- Cereal
- Oatmeal.

Beef
2-3 servings of lean protein
(1 serving = about 3 ounces/card size)
- Seafood
- Poultry.

Calcium and vitamin D

Low levels of calcium and vitamin D are associated with adverse maternal and infant health outcomes, but it is not clear whether low levels are a causal factor or a marker of poor maternal health.

The development of the fetal skeleton requires approximately 30 g of calcium during pregnancy, and this is mainly in the last trimester. This total amount is a relatively small percentage of the total calcium in the mother's body and can be easily mobilized from maternal stores if needed. Intestinal absorption and renal retention of calcium increase progressively during
during gestation.

For pregnant women with low baseline dietary calcium intake, high-dose calcium supplementation may reduce the risk of developing hypertension during pregnancy.

Examples of daily calcium sources include 3-4 servings of dairy products:
- milk (1 serving = 1 cup);
- eggs (1 serving = 1 large egg);
- yogurt (1 serving = 1 cup);
- pasteurized cheese (1 serving = approximately 1.5 ounces or the size of your hand);
- tofu (1 serving = ½ cup);
- white beans (1 serving = approximately ½ cup)
- almonds (1 serving = approximately ⅓ cup)
- salmon (1 serving = approximately 3 ounces);
- white beans (1 serving = approximately ½ cup);
- almonds (1 serving = approximately ⅓ cup);
- salmon (1 serving = approximately 3 ounces);

The recommended daily intake of calcium is 1000 to 1300 mg for pregnant and lactating women, depending on age.

Vitamin D.

In addition to its role in calcium and bone homeostasis, vitamin D may regulate many other cellular functions.

Poor vitamin D status in the perinatal period can have short- and long-term consequences for bones, the immune system, and overall health.

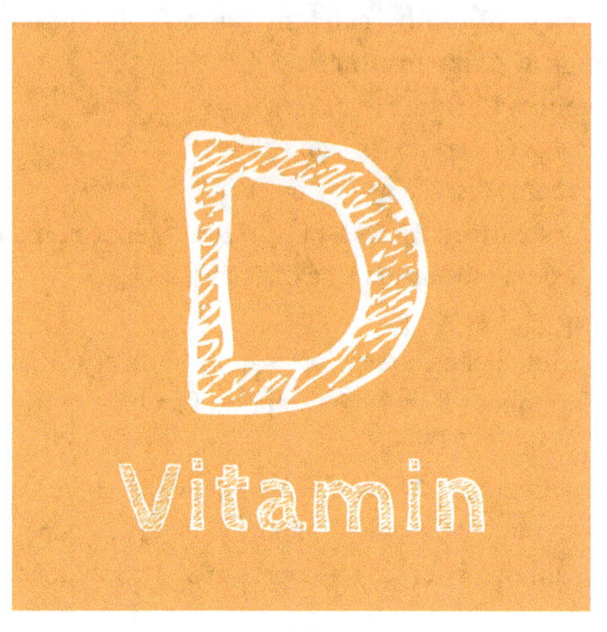

Dietary recommendations suggest a daily intake of 600 international units during pregnancy. According to statistics, vitamin D deficiency affects 40 to 98 percent of pregnant women worldwide.

Supplements often state the type of vitamin D they contain. Most prescription prenatal vitamins contain cholecalciferol (this is D3), but some contain ergocalciferol (this is D2), and some contain a mixture. Many commercial over-the-counter products labeled "vitamin D" (such as multivitamin supplements, fortified milk, and bread) contain D2. **D3 is more easily converted to active forms of**

vitamin D and is more effective at increasing serum 25-hydroxyvitamin D.

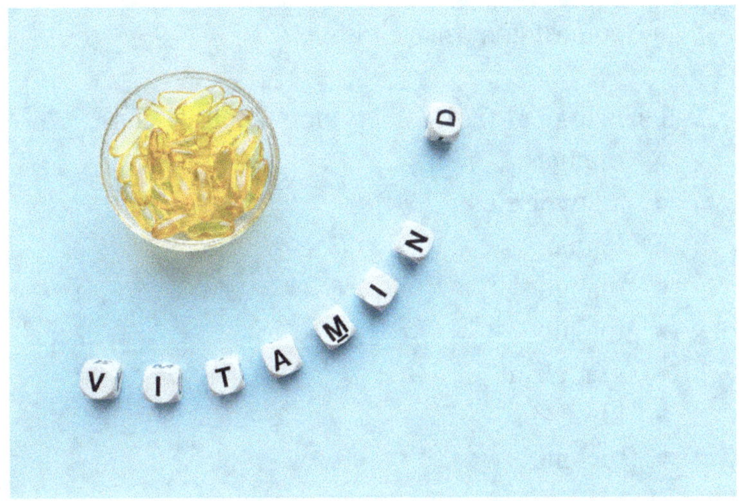

Skin synthesis after exposure to sunlight is the main natural source of the vitamin. **Very few foods contain vitamin D naturally, such as fish, eggs, especially chicken yolk, and wild mushrooms such as chanterelles.**

Folic acid is recommended at a dose of 0.6-0.8 mg/day for pregnant women.

Examples of daily sources of folic acid
2 servings of dark green leafy vegetables (1 serving = about 1 cup)

- beets
- spinach
- lettuce leaves;
- collard greens.

2-3 servings of fruit (1 serving = about ½ cup)
- oranges;
- strawberries
- lemon
- mango
- tomato
- grapefruit
- kiwi;
- melon.

3 servings of whole grains (1 serving = about ½ cup or 1 slice):
- bread
- corn flour
- cereal
- oatmeal.

2 servings of legumes (1 serving = about ½ cup):
- split peas
- red and white beans;
- black beans;
- navy beans
- black-eyed peas;

- chickpeas (garbanzo beans).

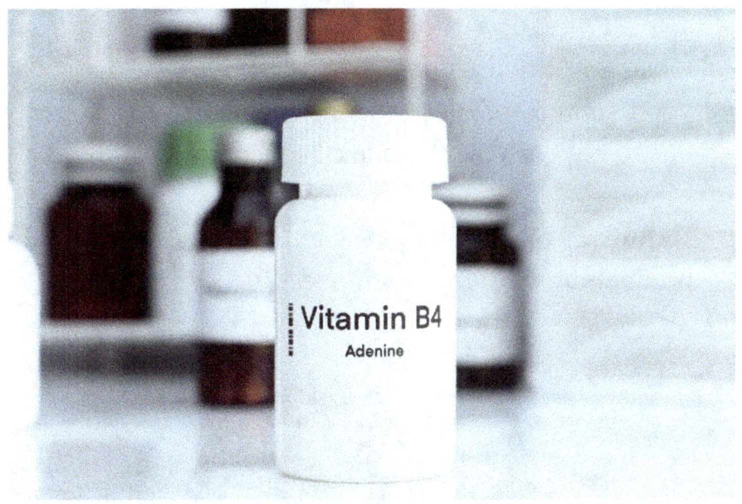

Choline is important for the development of the fetal central nervous system.

Pregnant women are **recommended to consume 450 mg/day, and its sources are in eggs, meat, poultry, seafood, and dairy products.** Plant sources, such as beans, Brussels sprouts, broccoli, and spinach, contain lower amounts of choline; therefore, vegetarians and vegans should seek additional sources of choline.

Zinc plays a role in many biological functions, including normal fetal growth and neuronal development, and the recommended **daily allowance is 11 to 12 mg during pregnancy.**

And food sources of zinc include meat, poultry, and some types of seafood (such as oysters, crabs, and lobsters). Whole grains, cereals, and legumes are also good sources of zinc, but the bioavailability is lower due to phytates that bind and reduce its absorption.

Iodine is an important mineral needed for the production of thyroid hormones.

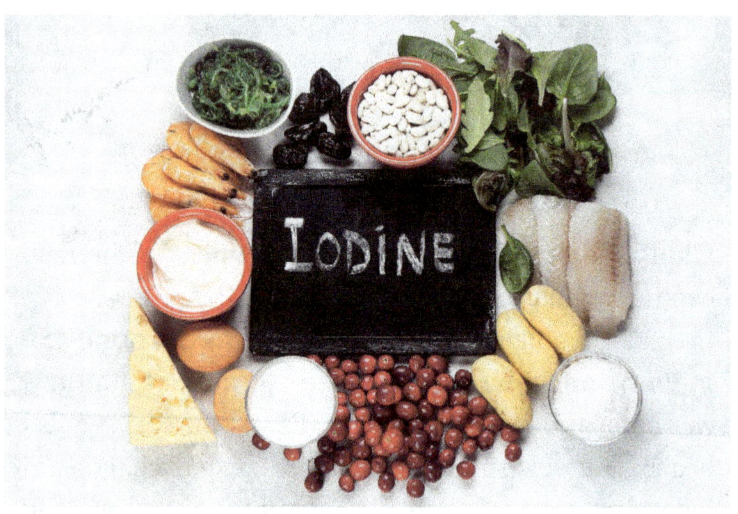

Iodine deficiency has potentially harmful effects, including maternal and fetal hypothyroidism. The National Academy of Medicine recommends an iodine intake of 220 mcg during pregnancy, and the WHO and the American Thyroid Association recommend a **daily iodine intake of 250 mcg** for both pregnant and breastfeeding mothers. Too much iodine can be harmful.

Many prenatal vitamins do not contain iodine, as the requirement is often met by dietary sources such as iodized salt. **Pregnant women should not be encouraged to start using table salt** if they have not already done so, but should be encouraged to use iodized salt.

Vitamin B12
Involved in DNA synthesis and cellular metabolism, the recommended daily intake during pregnancy is 2.6 mcg. **Sources include only animal products such as fish, meat, poultry, eggs, and dairy products.**

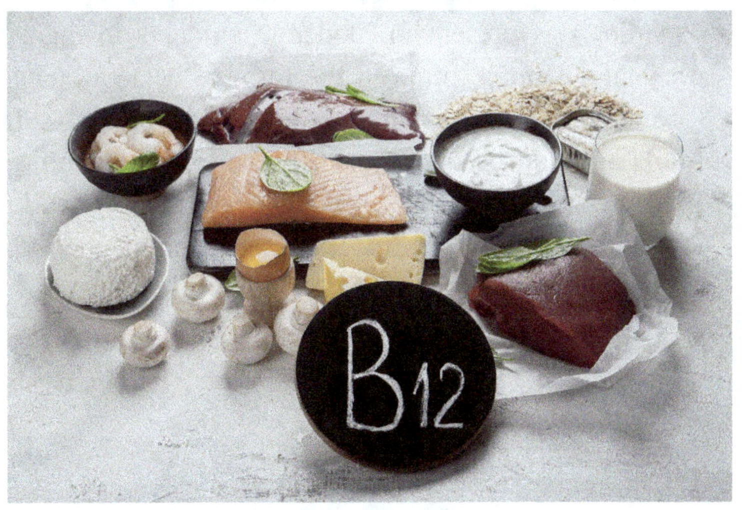

Vitamin A
Important for cell division, growth of fetal organs and skeleton, support of the immune system, development of fetal vision and support of maternal vision.

However, supplementation in patients without deficiency does not improve pregnancy outcomes and may increase the risk of toxicity. A pregnant woman with a moderate deficiency is at increased risk for hen-skin blindness, especially in the third trimester when fetal growth accelerates, because the fetus receives adequate vitamin A from maternal stores. The recommended intake of vitamin A increases to 750-770 mcg of retinol equivalents (i.e., 2500 to 2560 international units) during pregnancy.
Vitamin A is present in moderate amounts in many prenatal vitamins, often in the form of beta-carotene (provitamin A). **Vitamin A is found in a variety of foods and can be met by eating foods such as milk, fish, eggs, carrots, leafy greens, broccoli, cantaloupe, and zucchini.** It is also recommended to avoid eating liver due to its high vitamin A content.

Fluids:

During pregnancy, adequate fluid intake through beverage consumption (i.e., water and other liquids) is estimated to be about **5 pt lqd** (2.3 liters) **per day**.

Many factors (e.g., ambient temperature, humidity, physical activity and exertion) also affect total water requirements.

Fluoride.

Fluoride supplementation during pregnancy is unnecessary, even for pregnant women who live in areas where the water is not fluoridated.

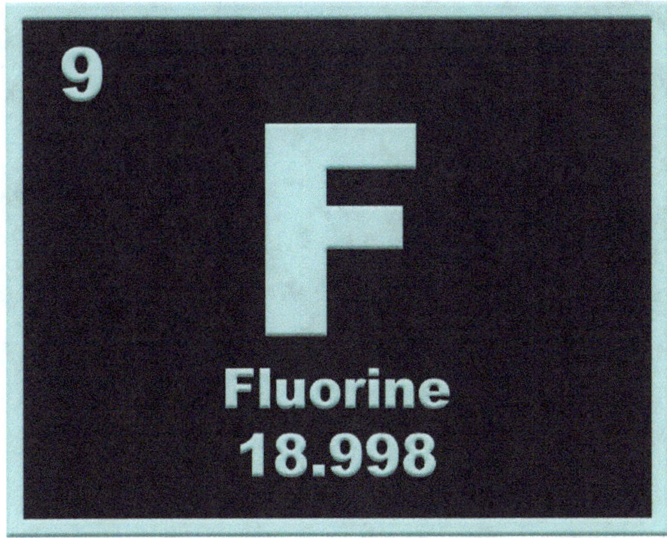

CHAPTER 3: CHOOSING THE RIGHT FOODS: VEGETABLES, FRUITS, CEREALS, MEAT, FISH, AND DAIRY PRODUCTS.

Gluten-free diet - Gluten-free grains often do not contain the same levels of added folic acid, calcium, and iron as wheat products; therefore, eliminating gluten-rich foods during pregnancy can lead to insufficient intake of these substances, as well as thiamine, riboflavin, and niacin.

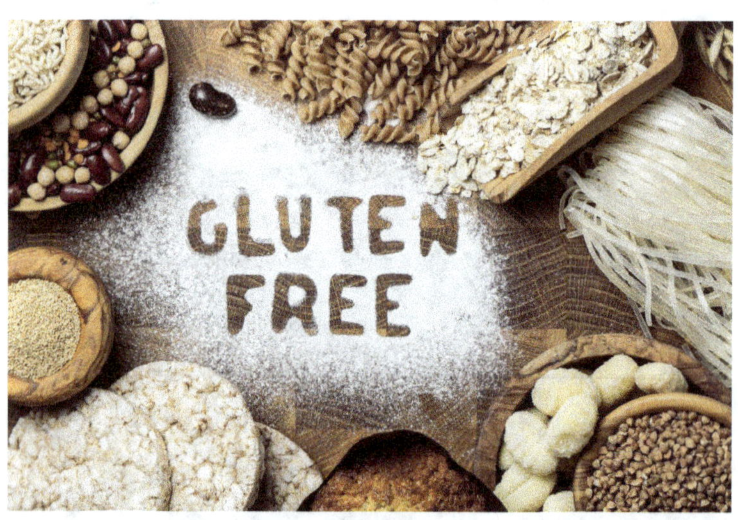

However, consumption of other whole grains (e.g., quinoa, brown rice, buckwheat, and gluten-free oats) in addition to standard folic acid supplements of 400

to 800 mcg/day should prevent deficiency, and under these conditions, these diets are considered safe.

Low carbohydrate diet

"Low-carb" diets vary greatly in terms of the amount of carbohydrates they consume. Technically, any diet that provides less than 45 percent of its energy from carbohydrates can be considered "low-carb." For a 2000-calorie diet, this would be less than 225 grams per day. It is recommended to avoid extremely low-carb diets during pregnancy. Moderate carbohydrate restriction may be acceptable, especially for pregnant women with gestational diabetes, but this should be done under supervision.

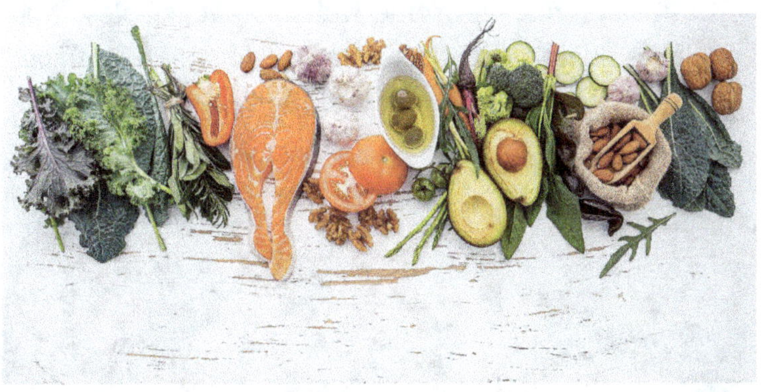

The ketogenic diet is a type of very low-carbohydrate diet that classically consists of high fat, moderate protein, and extremely low carbohydrate intake, which causes metabolic changes associated with a state of starvation.

Ketogenic diets typically limit carbohydrate intake to 5-10 percent of energy needs, which would provide only 25-50 grams of carbohydrate per day. There is minimal information on the effects of
 of a ketogenic diet on the fetus during pregnancy. Studies in rodents have reported potential adverse effects on the fetus, such as excessive fetal growth and changes in the size of organs and brain structures. **This diet is not recommended for use during pregnancy.**

Paleolithic Diet - This diet typically includes nuts, fish, meat, eggs, and some fruits and vegetables, and excludes dairy products, grains, legumes, refined sugars, table salt, and processed foods.

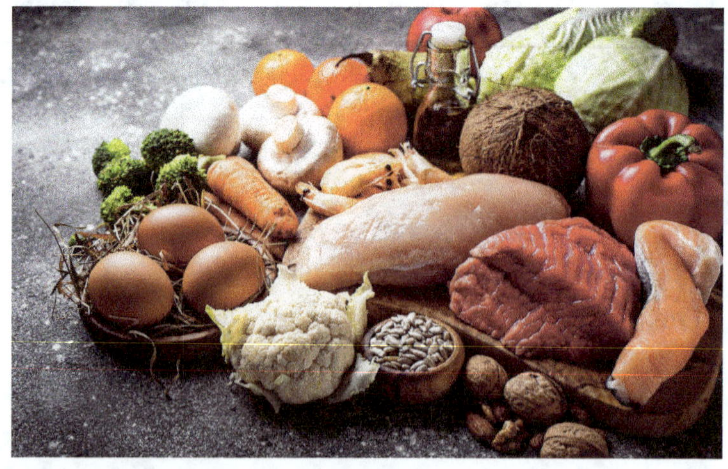

It is high in protein, moderate in fat (mostly unsaturated fat), low to moderate in carbohydrates, and low in sodium.

It may be low in folic acid, certain types of fiber, and calcium due to the exclusion of grains, legumes, and dairy products. There is little research on this diet for pregnant women, but a Paleo diet may be acceptable during pregnancy because it includes vegetables, fruits, and healthy proteins and eliminates or limits added sugars, certain processed foods, and processed meats.

However, it is important to remember that it does not provide adequate amounts of key nutrients. For pregnant women following the Paleo diet, a prenatal vitamin containing at least 400-800 micrograms of folic acid and 150-250 micrograms of iodine (if pregnant women do not use iodized table salt) is recommended, as well as calcium supplements of 1000 mg divided into 2-3 doses throughout the day. **Some sources do not recommend the Paleo diet because of the dairy restrictions.**

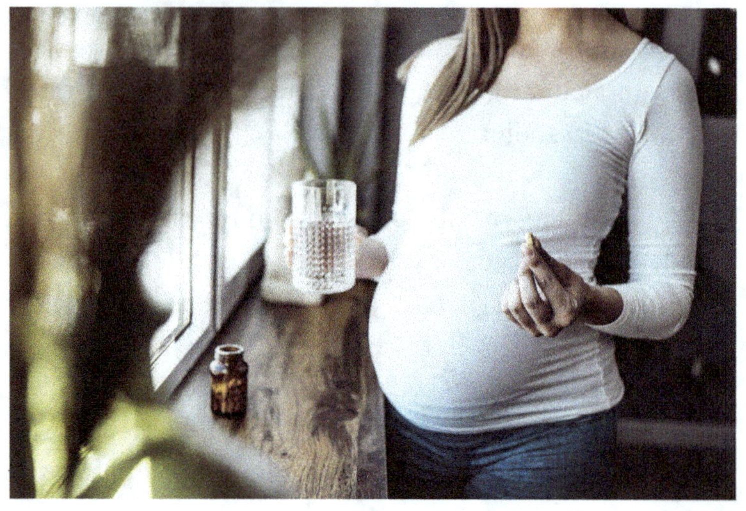

Intermittent fasting - this can include fasting for a few hours during the day or for one or more days. Fasting can be done for religious reasons or to promote weight loss. Unfortunately, the effects of intermittent fasting in healthy pregnant women are also poorly understood.

Fasting in Ramadan is about abstaining from food and drink during daylight hours during the month of Ramadan, and it is a religious practice followed by 30 to 85 percent of pregnant Muslim women, every professional may encounter this situation and should be prepared. This type of diet is also not fully understood, but there are studies that indicate that there are bad consequences of this diet.

Lactose intolerance. Pregnant women with lactose intolerance who cannot consume enough calcium through dairy products and other dietary components can take calcium supplements or consume calcium-fortified foods and beverages, such as soy-fortified drinks.

However, it should be noted that pregnant women with lactose digestion disorders improved their lactose tolerance in late pregnancy. This is due to the slowing of intestinal transit during pregnancy and the adaptation of bacteria to increased lactose intake.

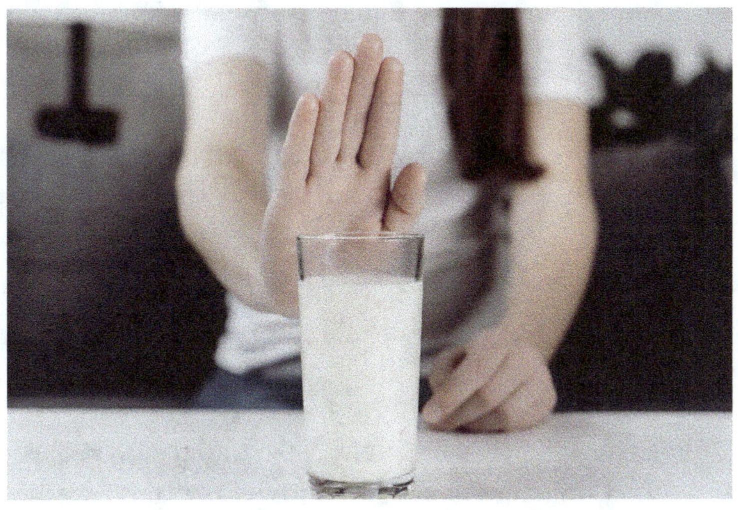

Products.

Fish:

Do not eat fish with a high mercury content, for example:
- Swordfish
- Tilefish
- King mackerel
- Shark.

Mercury is a metal whose high levels can harm your unborn child's brain - even before conception. Most of the time, mercury enters our bodies when we eat large predatory fish.

However, many types of seafood contain little or no mercury. Therefore, the risk of mercury exposure also depends on the amount and type of seafood you eat.

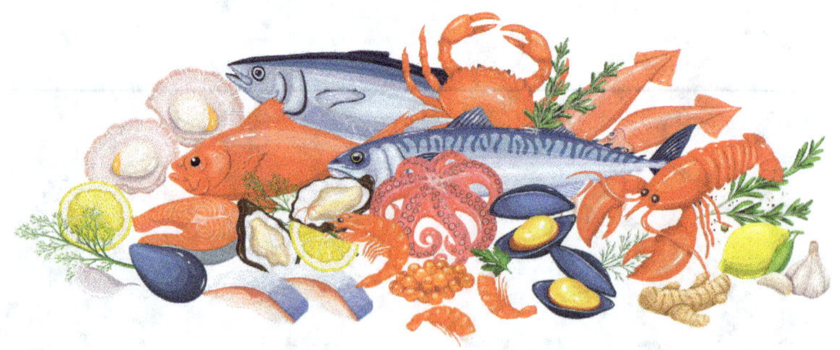

Pregnant women can safely eat a variety of cooked seafood, but they should not forget that they should avoid fish with a high mercury content. **It should be borne in mind that removing all fish from the diet will deprive you of important omega-3 fatty acids.**

Types of fish that are or are not suitable for consumption by pregnant and lactating mothers (by mercury content)

- Anchovy is the best choice
- Atlantic humpback is the best choice
- Atlantic mackerel - the best choice
- Black Sea bass - the best choice
- Bluefish - good choice
- Buffalo - good choice
- Oil fish - best choice
- Carp - good selection
- Catfish - best choice
- Chilean sea bass/Patagonian snapper - good choice
- Shellfish - best choice
- Cod - best choice
- Crab - best choice
- Crayfish - best choice
- Flounder (sea tongue) - best choice
- Perch - the best choice
- Haddock- the best choice
- Hake - the best choice
- Halibut - the best choice
- Herring- best choice

- King mackerel- avoid
- Lobster- best choice
- Mahi mahi / dolphin fish- good choice
- Marlin - avoid
- Sea devil - a good choice
- Mullet - better choice
- Orange roughy - avoid
- Oyster - better choice
- Pacific mackerel - better choice
- Freshwater bass - best choice
- Ocean perch - best choice
- Pickerel - best choice
- Pollock - the best choice
- Sea fish - good choice
- Sablefish - good choice
- Canned salmon - the best choice
- Fresh salmon - best choice
- Fresh/frozen salmon - best choice
- Sardine - best choice
- Scallop - best choice
- Shad - best choice
- Shark - avoid
- Cape crucian carp (sheep's head)
- Shrimp - better choice
- Smelt - best choice
- Snapper (Lucian) - good choice
- Spanish mackerel - better choice
- Squid - the best choice

- Striped bass (ocean) - best choice
- Swordfish - avoid
- Tilapia - better choice
- Tilefish (from the Gulf of Mexico) - avoid
- Shingles (from the Atlantic Ocean) - best choice
- Freshwater trout - best choice
- Tuna, albacore / white - good choice
- Tuna, canned - good choice
- Tuna, fresh/frozen - best choice
- Tuna, bigeye - avoid
- Tuna, light, canned - best choice
- Tuna, yellowfin - good choice
- Weak fish/trout - good choice
- White humpback / Pacific - good choice
- Humpback whiting - good choice
- Whitefish - the best choice
- Whitefish - the best choice

Grain.
Bread, pasta, oatmeal, cereal, and tortillas are all grain products. Whole grains are those that have not been processed and include the kernel of the whole grain. **Oats, barley, quinoa, brown rice, and bulgur are whole grains, as are products made from these grains.** Look for the words "whole grain" on the product label, and make half of your grain servings whole grains.

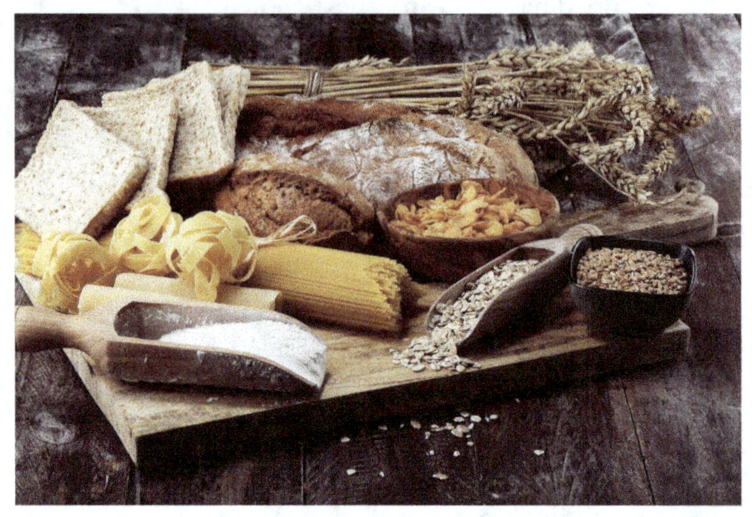

What kinds of fruit should a pregnant woman eat?
A pregnant woman can eat fresh fruit as well as canned, frozen, or dried fruit. Juice, which is 100% fruit juice, counts as fruit, but it is best to eat mostly whole fruit instead of juice. Aim for half a plate of fruits and vegetables at each meal.

What kinds of vegetables should a pregnant woman eat?
She can eat raw, canned, frozen, or dried vegetables or drink 100% vegetable juice. Dairy products that a pregnant woman eats should be pasteurized, skimmed, or low-fat varieties.

Foods and vitamins:
Vegetables such as carrots, sweet potatoes, squash, spinach, cooked greens, tomatoes, and red peppers are good sources of vitamin A and potassium. **Fruits:** Melons, nectarines, mangoes, prunes, bananas, apricots, oranges, and red or pink grapefruit are also good sources of potassium. **Dairy products**, such as low-fat yogurt, skim milk, or soy milk, are good sources of calcium, potassium, and vitamins A and D.

And grains:
ready-to-eat cereals and cooked porridge for iron and folic acid.

In addition to main meals, you should have snacks. Choose healthy snacks, for example:
- Low-fat or fat-free yogurt with fruit (but look for options without added sugar).
- Whole grain crackers with peanut butter.
- A carrot or fruit platter.

CHAPTER 4: VEGETARIAN DIETS

The nutritional adequacy of a vegetarian diet should be evaluated on an individual basis, based on the type, amount, and variety of nutrients a person consumes. Specifically, a healthy vegetarian diet includes the same amount of vegetables, fruits, and dairy products as a healthy regular diet.

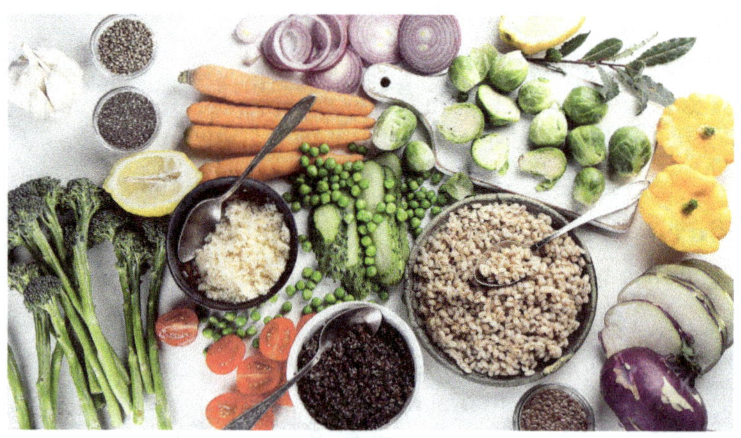

To compensate for the lack of meat, poultry, and seafood, the amount of grains should be increased by half a cup per day, with an increase in vegetarian protein sources: nuts and seeds, soy products, beans/peas/lentils, and eggs.

Vegetarian diets have many subtypes and are often grouped in order from less restrictive to more restrictive, with subtypes:

- **Semi-vegetarians** are people who occasionally eat meat, fish, or chicken in their diet. Some people who follow this diet may not eat red meat, but may eat fish and possibly chicken. In some Asian cultures, animal protein sources may be consumed only once or twice a week.

- **Pescetarians** are vegetarians whose diet sometimes includes fish in addition to eggs, milk, and dairy products, but does not include other animal meat.

- **Lacto-ovo-vegetarianism** - consists of the inclusion of eggs, milk and dairy products (from the words lacto- = dairy; ovo- = eggs), but this diet does not include meat. This type of diet may result in insufficient intake of omega-3 fatty acids.

- **Lacto-vegetarianism** - the diet includes milk and dairy products, but does not include eggs and meat. This diet may result in insufficient intake of choline and omega-3 fatty acids, and possible insufficient intake of iron.

- **Macrobiotics** - emphasizes whole grain products, especially brown rice, and the diet includes vegetables, fruits, legumes and seaweed. Local fruits are also recommended. Animal products, limited to white meat or white fish, can be included in the diet once or twice a week. This diet may have insufficient intake of vitamin B12, choline, iron, calcium, and omega-3 fatty acids.

- **Vegan type** - here, all animal products are excluded from the diet, including eggs, milk, and dairy products. Some vegans also don't eat honey. They may also avoid foods that are processed or not organically grown. This type of diet may result in insufficient intake of vitamin B12, choline, iron, calcium, and omega-3 fatty acids.

Potential problems with these diets include:

Low birth weight and short stature for gestational age. Some studies have reported this among pregnant women following a vegetarian or vegan diet. Insufficient intake of micronutrients. Well-balanced vegetarian diets are similar to a well-balanced diet because they meet most nutrients, with the exception of iron, vitamin D, vitamin E, and choline for some types of vegetarian diets. n B12 and omega-3 fatty acids.

Other nutrients of potential concern, especially for vegans and diets that completely eliminate animal products, include calcium, vitamin B12, and omega-3 fatty acids.

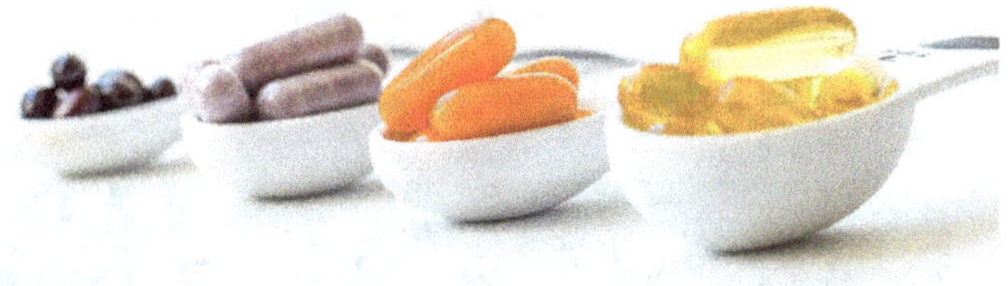

If all animal foods are excluded and dietary modification is not possible or likely, one or more of the following supplements should be considered, these are:
- Vitamin B12
- Omega-3 fatty acids (e.g. vegan algae supplements)
- Choline
- Iron
- Vitamin D

- Vitamin E
- Calcium

Insufficient consumption of macronutrients

Limited studies of populations outside the United States have shown that macronutrient intakes of pregnant vegetarians were similar to vegetarians, except that pregnant vegetarians consumed statistically less protein and more carbohydrates; however, no studies have reported protein deficiencies in pregnant vegetarians.

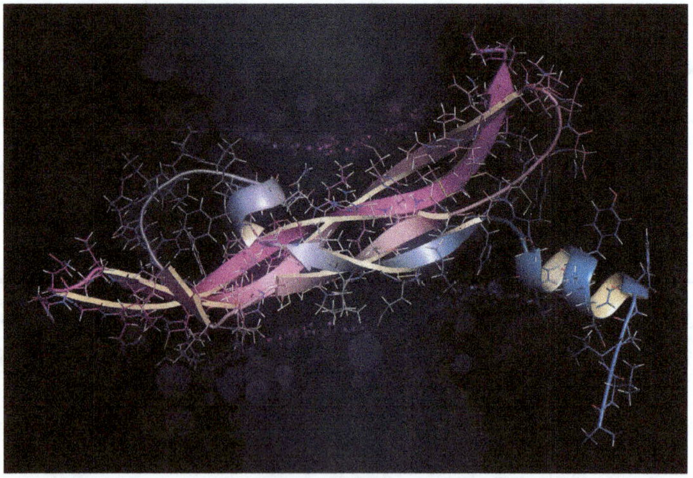

The quality of protein in a well-balanced diet should be of concern if the total energy intake is adequate (as it provides a protein storage effect). Protein is made up of amino acids, including the nine essential amino acids that our body cannot produce on its own.

Animal foods have about twice as much protein per serving (about 0.7oz (20 g)) as plant foods (which have 0.35oz (10g) or less).

And unlike animal foods, plant foods do not contain all nine essential amino acids. That's why it's important to get your protein from a variety of vegetarian sources, ideally including a protein meal at every meal.

Good sources of plant-based protein include
- Eggs.
- Dairy products.
- Legumes, such as chickpeas, beans, and lentils.
- Soy products, including tempeh, tofu, soy milk, and soy beans.

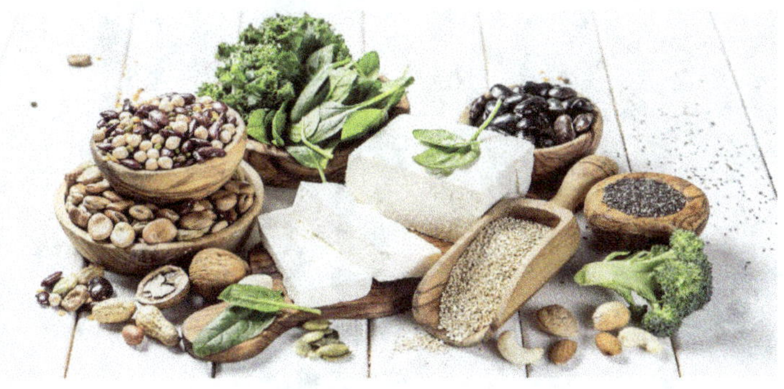

- Many nuts, seeds, and nut butters (such as peanuts, almonds, cashews, chia seeds, flax seeds, and walnuts).

And for vegans, it can be tofu, lentils, beans, nutritional yeast, green peas, soy milk, nuts, oatmeal, and spirulina.

If not vitamin supplements, what other foods can be added?

Iron in the diet of pregnant women:
Iron supports the physical growth and neurological development of the baby. It also improves circulation in the pregnant woman, which is especially important now that blood volume increases by 20-100% during pregnancy.
In fact, iron deficiency is the most common nutritional deficiency during pregnancy.

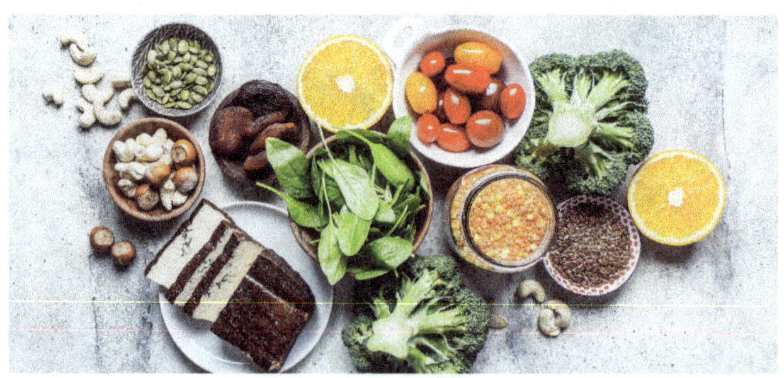

A pregnant woman's prenatal vitamin can meet some of her iron needs, but she should eat several servings of a variety of iron-rich foods each day.

Good sources of iron include

- Iron-fortified breakfast cereals.
- Beans and other legumes.
- Tofu, tempeh, and other soy foods.
- Whole-grain or fortified foods, such as bread and pasta.
- Dark leafy vegetables, such as spinach, kale, and Swiss chard.
- Dark chocolate.
- Dark green vegetables.
- Dried fruits, such as apricots.

Vegetable foods contain non-heme iron, which is more difficult for our bodies to absorb than heme iron, which is found in animal foods.

Avoid drinking tea or coffee with meals, as this can make it more difficult for the body to absorb iron from vegetables. It is advisable to combine iron-rich foods with something rich in vitamin C, such as orange juice, tomato sauce, or broccoli.

Vitamin B12
Pregnant women need 2.6 micrograms daily.

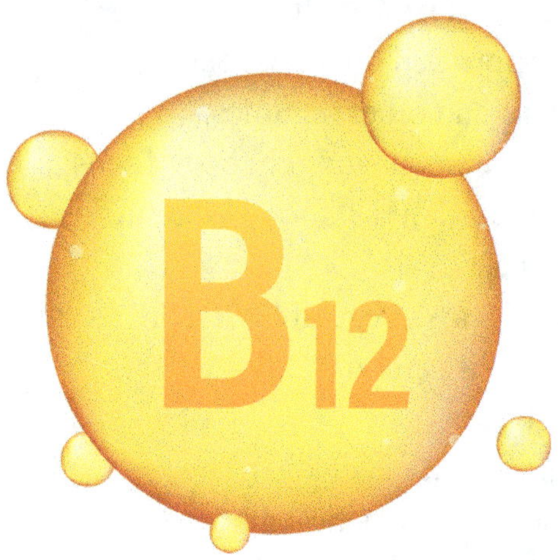

It plays an important role in the development of your baby's brain and is naturally found only in animal foods. Eating several servings of dairy products a day should provide a pregnant woman with enough.

When it comes to vegans, they need to eat foods fortified with vitamin B12, such as
- Soy and other vegetable milks;
- Dry breakfast cereals;
- nutritional yeast.

And for vegetarians, it also includes milk, cheese, and eggs.

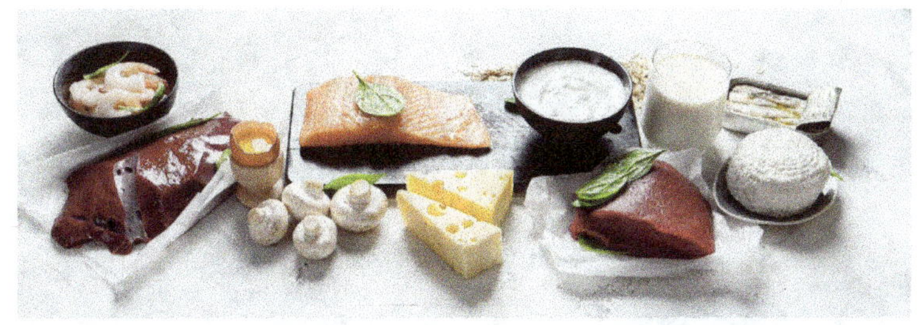

Vitamin D

This vitamin helps the body absorb calcium to support the development of the child's bones. Fatty fish is the best source, but not in the case of our diets.

Vegetarian food sources are enriched with vitamin D:
- egg yolk;
- some breakfast cereals and fatty spreads;
- some types of tofu;
- orange juice.

Vitamin D is found in only a small number of foods, making it difficult to get enough from foods that naturally contain vitamin D and from fortified foods alone.

That's why all adults, including non-pregnant women, should consider taking a daily supplement.

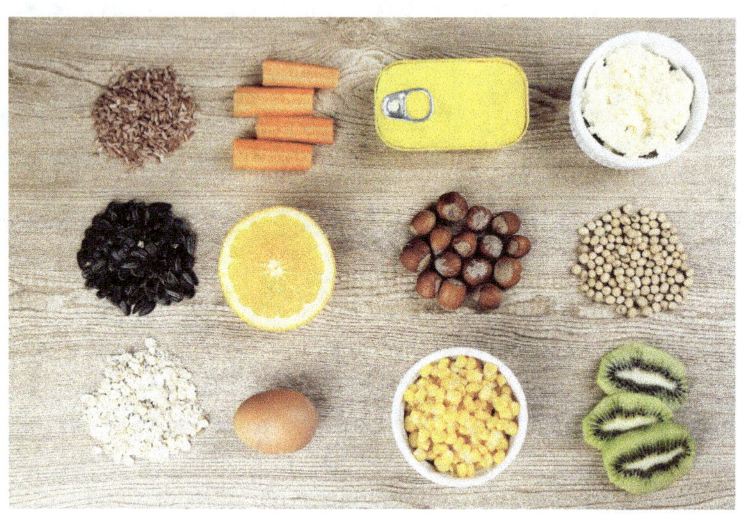

Calcium.

Calcium builds a baby's bones and helps protect a pregnant woman's bones. In fact, what the baby doesn't get from the food the pregnant woman eats, she gets from her bones, especially in the last trimester, which increases the risk of osteoporosis.

One serving of most dairy products and fortified soy milk provides about one-third of the daily calcium requirement, and the daily dose is 1000 mg. Other fortified foods and plant foods on the list contain about 100 mg of calcium (or less) per serving.

As a pregnant woman, include several servings of the following foods in your diet each day:

- Milk, cheese, and yogurt.
- Calcium-fortified almond or soy milk, orange juice, and breakfast cereals.
- White beans, chickpeas and lentils.
- Sesame seeds, almonds and tahini.
- Dried figs.
- Tofu containing calcium (look for calcium chloride or sulfate in the list of ingredients).
- Certain green vegetables, including cabbage, turnip greens, mustard greens, broccoli, and bok choy (others, such as spinach and beet greens, contain calcium, but our bodies don't absorb calcium from these vegetables either).
- Dried fruits.

Iodine.

Iodine helps the pregnant woman's thyroid gland to produce certain hormones and is crucial for the development of the fetus' brain and central nervous system. Too low iodine levels can lead to hypothyroidism or goiter.

Good sources of iodine for vegetarians include cow's milk, seaweed, iodized table salt, dairy products, and eggs.

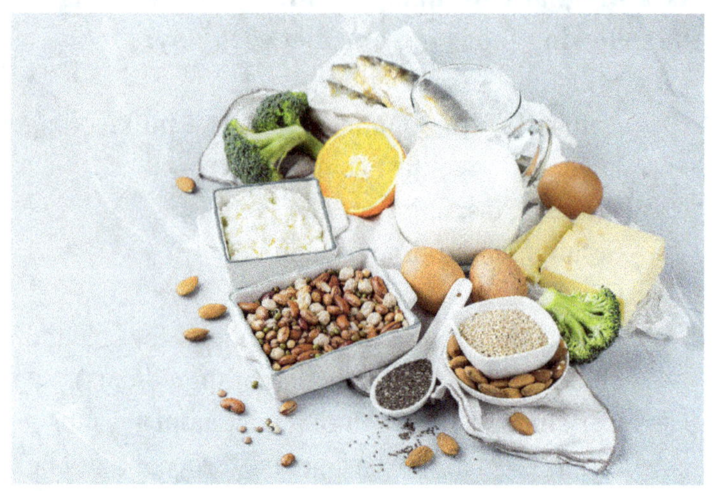

Iodine can also be found in plant foods, such as grains, but its level depends on the amount of iodine in the soil where it is grown.

You need 220 micrograms per day.

Zinc

Zinc - 11 mg per day.

Zinc supports growth during pregnancy, and a pregnant woman will need a constant supply of it because her body has no way to store it.

The best source of zinc is animal foods, as the human body does not absorb zinc from plant foods as efficiently.

Good sources of zinc include:

- Fortified breakfast cereals.
- Beans.

- Whole grain products.
- Nuts and seeds.
- Oatmeal.
- Milk, yogurt and cheese.

Folic acid is necessary for:
cell growth; and also reduces the likelihood of neural tube defects. You need about 400-800 micrograms per day, foods: dark leafy green vegetables, wheat germ, beans, and orange juice.

Omega 3
Omega 3 fatty acids, 200 mg per day Omega-3 contributes to the development of the baby's eyes and brain during pregnancy. Some studies also show that it can help reduce the risk of premature birth. It is found in fish, fish oil and microalgae.
Some yogurts, soy drinks, and juices are also fortified with Omega-3. But by far the easiest way for

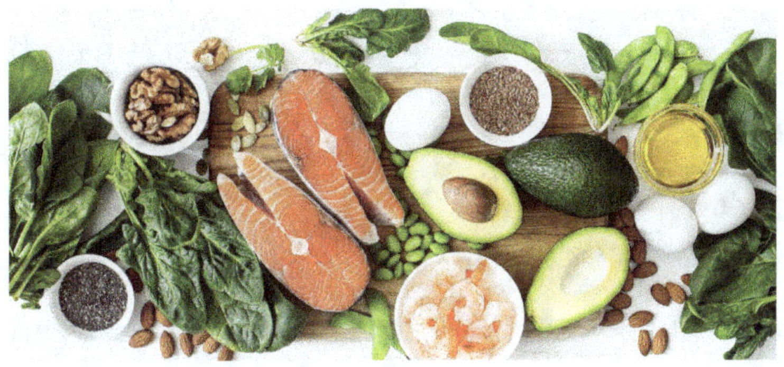

vegetarians to get the recommended dose is to take an algae-derived omega-3 supplement.

Is it safe to have a vegetarian or vegan pregnancy?

Whether a pregnant woman is vegetarian or vegan, she can have a healthy pregnancy with proper planning. As long as she eats a variety of healthy vegetarian foods and includes the key nutrients needed for the development of her baby's cells, brain, and organs, she can get all the nutrition she needs without meat, fish, or poultry (and of course also without animal products such as eggs and dairy if she is vegan).

In fact, a well-designed plant-based diet is rich in nutrients that support infant development and maternal health, including high levels of fiber, vitamins, and minerals. Therefore, a major task in working with pregnant vegetarians is to properly formulate their diet so that there are no deficiencies of

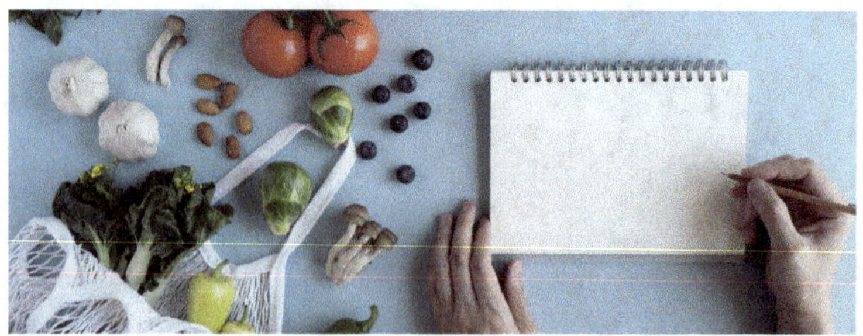

important components, as well as to add vitamin supplements in a timely manner.

EXAMPLES OF BALANCED VEGETARIAN AND VEGAN MEALS

Vegan or vegetarian breakfast for pregnant women
- Top with yogurt, soy yogurt or cottage cheese with berries and chia seeds.
- Break eggs and mix with beans and sautéed tomatoes.
- Make a tofu scramble with dark leafy greens.
- Eat fortified cereals (check for iron, zinc B12) with calcium-fortified soymilk.

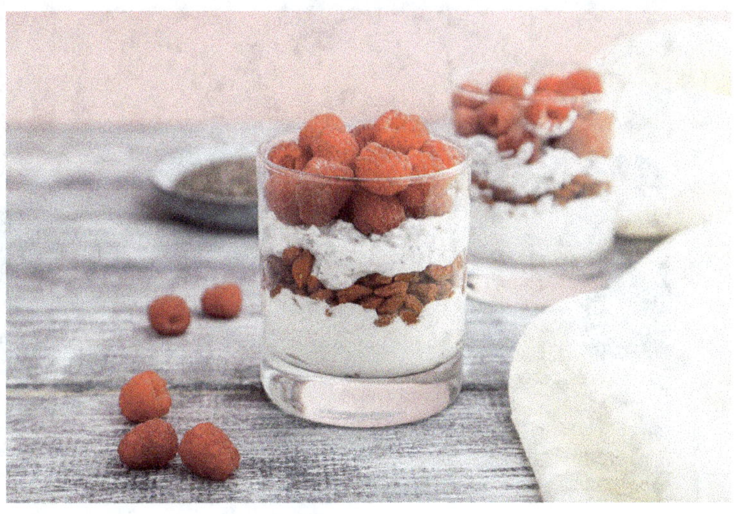

Vegan or vegetarian lunches and dinners for pregnant women

- Add beans (e.g. black or white), chickpeas, lentils or diced tofu to a green salad.
- Fill a bag with black beans or hummus and chopped raw vegetables.
- Slice a hard-boiled egg and add to the sandwich.
- Drizzle tahini on the falafel sandwich.
- Chop tempeh and use as a base for tacos, enchiladas, or pasta sauce.
- Marinate tempeh or tofu and stir-fry with bok choy, broccoli, and other vegetables. Serve over whole grain rice.

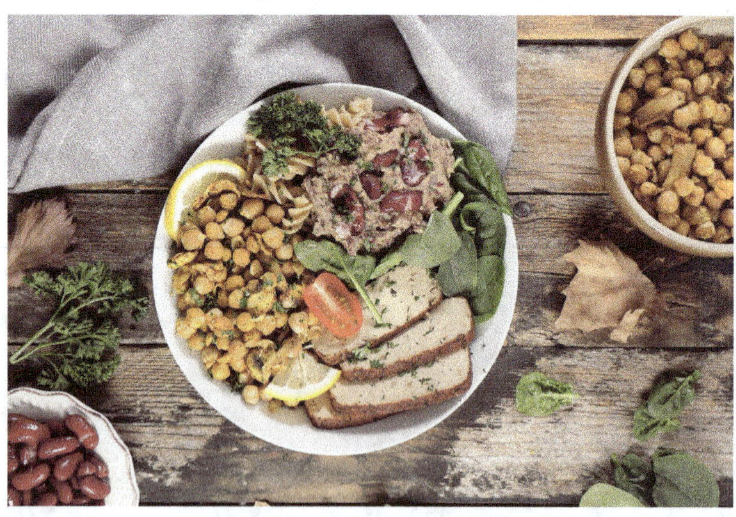

Vegan or vegetarian snack ideas for pregnancy

- Snack on a handful of almonds, walnuts, cashews, sunflower seeds, or roasted chickpeas.
- Spread peanut butter or almond butter on whole grain bread or sliced apples.
- Make chia pudding with fortified plant milk.
- Blend a smoothie with fruit, fortified plant milk, and nut butter.
- Dip raw vegetables and whole grain chips in hummus.

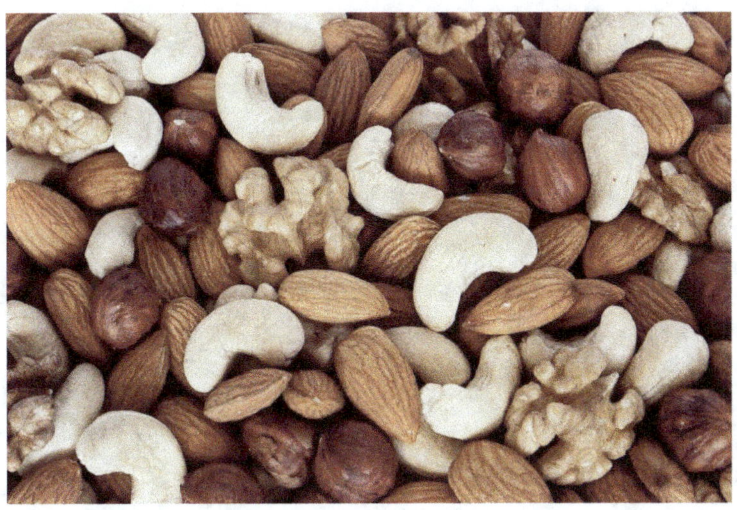

CHAPTER 5: GESTATIONAL DIABETES MELLITUS

What is gestational diabetes mellitus?

This is a disorder of carbohydrate metabolism, namely an increase in plasma glucose levels, which first occurred in a woman during pregnancy. Signs of gestational diabetes accompany the 2-3 trimester. The disease disappears on its own after childbirth.

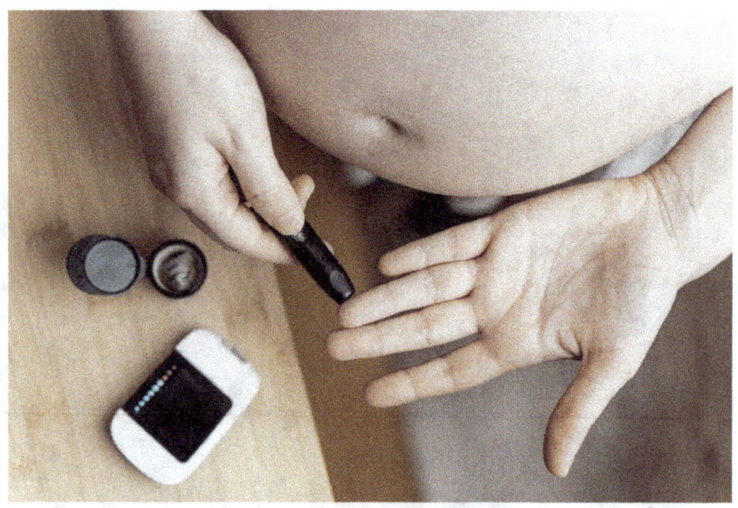

The tactic is therapeutic dietary therapy.

Dietary goals:

- To achieve normoglycemia.
- Prevention of ketosis.
- Ensuring adequate nutrition.
- Ensuring adequate weight gain during pregnancy
- during pregnancy based on the mother's body mass index.
- Promoting fetal well-being.

A balanced diet means eating a variety of healthy foods. If the pregnant woman is a vegetarian or follows a special diet, you need to make sure she gets a balanced diet.

What should you eat?

- Plenty of whole fruits and vegetables.
- Moderate amounts of lean protein and healthy fats.
- Moderate amounts of whole grains, such as bread, cereal, pasta, and rice, and starchy vegetables, such as corn and peas.
- Fewer foods high in sugar, such as
- soft drinks, fruit juices, and pastries.

Pregnant women with gestational diabetes should eat three small to medium-sized meals and several snacks each day. Do not skip meals or snacks. Keep the amount of food you eat about the same each day. This can help keep blood glucose levels stable.

In addition, walking, swimming, or other low-impact exercise may be recommended because exercise can help control blood glucose levels.

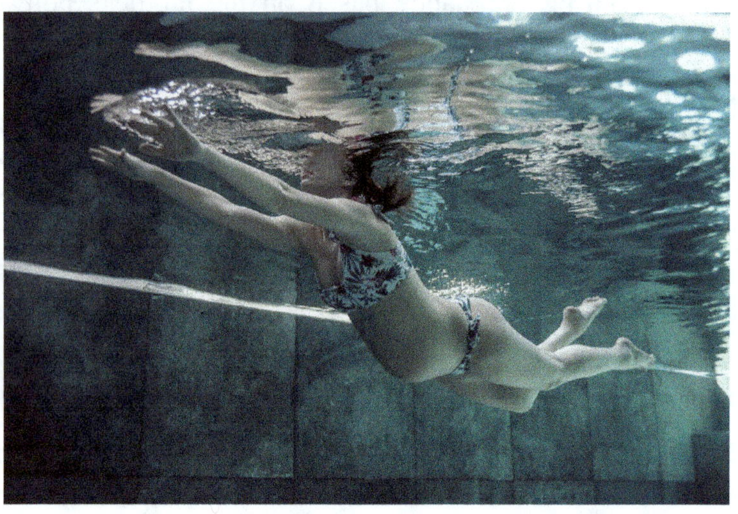

The caloric needs of pregnant women with gestational diabetes are the same as those of pregnant women without diabetes. After calculating caloric needs, carbohydrate intake is determined because it is the main nutrient that affects postprandial glucose levels. The rise in postprandial glucose levels can be suppressed by limiting carbohydrates in the diet. However, reducing carbohydrate intake to lower postprandial glucose levels may result in increased fat intake, which can negatively affect maternal insulin resistance and fetal body composition.

The main thing to remember is to focus on slow, healthy carbohydrates with a low glycemic index! The rest of your calories should come from protein and fat. Protein intake should be spread throughout the day and included in all meals and snacks to promote satiety, slow the absorption of carbohydrates into the bloodstream, and provide enough calories.
A high-protein snack is recommended before bedtime to prevent accelerated (i.e., hunger) ketosis during the night and to maintain fasting (i.e., hunger) glucose levels within the target range.

Recommendations:
- Eat regularly - usually three meals a day + snacks;
- Eat starchy foods with a low glycemic index that release sugar slowly, such as whole grain pasta, brown rice, whole grain breads, bran cereals, legumes, beans, lentils, granola, and plain cereals;
- Eat lots of fruits and vegetables - aim for at least 5 servings a day;
- Avoid sugary foods - a sugar-free diet is not required, but snacks such as cakes and cookies

should be replaced with healthier alternatives such as fruits, nuts and seeds;
- Avoid sugary drinks - diet drinks or sugar-free drinks are better than sugary drinks. Fruit juices and smoothies can also contain a lot of sugar, as can some drinks without added sugar, so it's worth checking the nutrition label;
- Eat lean sources of protein.

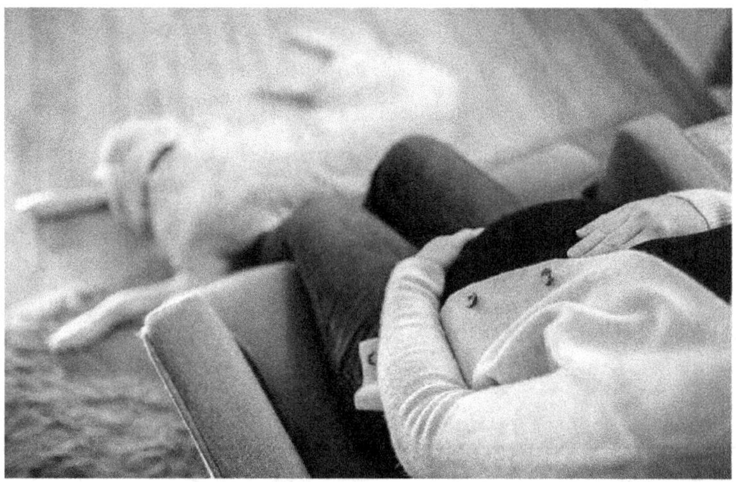

Pregnancy toxicosis is a common condition among pregnant women that manifests itself with nausea, vomiting, hypersensitivity to odors, and salivation (sialorrhea).

There is a very good question - **why does pregnancy toxicity occur and how can it be treated?**

In fact, there are many theories, and although none of them has been reliably confirmed, there are three most common opinions:
- First, during pregnancy, the amount of progesterone increases, which is known to decrease intestinal motility, and as a result, pregnant women experience all the "wonderful" symptoms of pregnancy.
- Second, there is also the effect of an increase in the amount of B-hCG and estrogen.
- Thirdly, the genetic factor also plays an important role.

Nausea during pregnancy can occur at any time of the day or night. Since nearly 75% of women experience morning sickness, there are many proven and reliable nutritional methods for relief. For some women, it is very important to consume certain foods in advance to treat morning sickness. Other expectant mothers find relief with certain foods and drinks right when the nausea begins.
It is also important to eat and drink after vomiting to replace fluids, electrolytes, and calories.

This means that you can have a snack in the morning before you get out of bed, like a banana on your nightstand, or have snacks at night that can also be helpful, like peanut butter crackers or cheese.

And these are the foods and drinks that can help manage nausea during pregnancy:
- Soft, easily digested foods (bananas, rice, applesauce, toast).
- Cold drinks and snacks (smoothies or almond milk)
- Ginger.
- Carbonated drinks.
- Herbal decoctions.
- Fruits and vegetables high in water (watermelon and cucumbers).
- Citrus fruits.
- Peppermint.
- Foods high in vitamin B6 (salmon and avocados).

Experts have found that protein-rich foods can help manage nausea during pregnancy.
Proteins such as chicken, peanut butter, and beans can calm waves of nausea by increasing a hormone called gastrin, which aids digestion. Other high-protein foods that help with morning sickness

are hard-boiled eggs, hard cheeses, nuts, lean beef, and Greek yogurt.

Hot food and drinks often have a flavor that triggers the gag reflex.

The olfactory system needs warmth to recognize an odor, so the warmer something is, the stronger it smells. Cold foods have less flavor, so they can be more enjoyable when you feel nauseous during pregnancy.

Great options are chilled almond milk, which can also soothe heartburn, or smoothies, which contain healthy fruits and are good for pregnant women.

If it is difficult to keep fluids down, you should try frozen yogurt, ice cream, or chilled fruit.

What other tips can there be?

And these are the foods and drinks that can help manage nausea during pregnancy:

- Eat meals and snacks slowly and in small portions every one to two hours to avoid stretching your stomach, which can make nausea worse in some women. Rinsing your mouth with water, brushing your teeth, or sucking on mints can reduce nausea after eating.
- Determine which foods they tolerate best and advise them to consume those foods.

- Consume liquids at least 30 minutes before or after solid foods to minimize the feeling of fullness in the stomach.
- Choose cold (or partially frozen), clear, carbonated, or acidic liquids. Sea ice cream and ginger ale are often well tolerated. However, some patients do not tolerate carbonated beverages well, as the release of carbon dioxide can cause stomach distension and exacerbate symptoms. Some patients find flavored liquids, such as lemon or mint tea, more favorable and helpful in reducing nausea.
- Consume liquids in small amounts; using a straw or a very small cup sometimes helps.
- Avoiding triggers is an important measure to reduce symptoms along with dietary changes.
- Examples of some triggers include: stuffy rooms, odors (e.g., perfume, chemicals, food, smoke), heat, humidity, noise, and visual or physical movement (e.g., flashing lights, driving). Lying down immediately after a meal and lying on the left side are potentially aggravating factors, as these actions can delay stomach emptying. Rapid changes in body position and insufficient rest can also aggravate symptoms.

CHAPTER 6: GASTROESOPHAGEAL REFLUX (HEARTBURN)

Gastroesophageal reflux (abbreviated as GERD or heartburn) is observed in 40 to 85% of pregnant women. Most studies describe an increase in the prevalence of symptoms from the first to the third trimester, with relief after delivery.

Although GERD symptoms can be severe, erosive gastropathy and other complications are rare. And GERD, unfortunately, tends to recur during subsequent pregnancies.

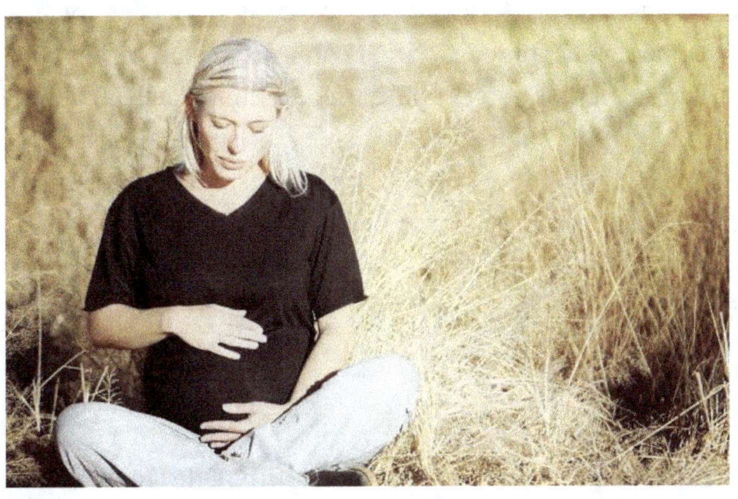

The pathogenesis of GERD during pregnancy involves both mechanical and internal factors that negatively affect the tone of the lower esophageal sphincter.

Lower esophageal sphincter pressure is below the lower limit of normal in all trimesters and returns to normal in the postpartum period.

The initial treatment for gastroesophageal reflux disease during pregnancy is lifestyle and dietary changes (e.g., raising the head of the bed and avoiding food triggers).

Sleeping on your left side may also help.

Patients with persistent GERD should be started on medication, but this will be done by a doctor.

Foods that cause symptoms should be avoided because some foods cause relaxation of the lower esophageal sphincter, which can lead to acid reflux.

These include excessive caffeine, chocolate, alcohol, soda, peppermint, and fatty, spicy, or acidic foods.

If you notice that your symptoms get worse after consuming certain foods or drinks (i.e., trigger foods), it is advisable to limit or avoid these things. There is also advice about portions, it is better to eat small meals.

Stop smoking.

In principle, this should be done in spite of GERD. But if you look at it from the reflux side, the fact is that saliva helps neutralize the acid that is released, and smoking reduces the amount of saliva in the mouth and throat. Smoking also reduces the pressure in the lower esophageal sphincter and provokes coughing, causing frequent episodes of acid reflux in the esophagus.

Avoid late meals

Lying down with a full stomach can increase the risk of acid reflux. Eating at least two to three hours before bedtime can help reduce symptoms. This is especially true for people with nocturnal reflux. Sit up straight during and immediately after eating. This relieves pressure on the abdomen.

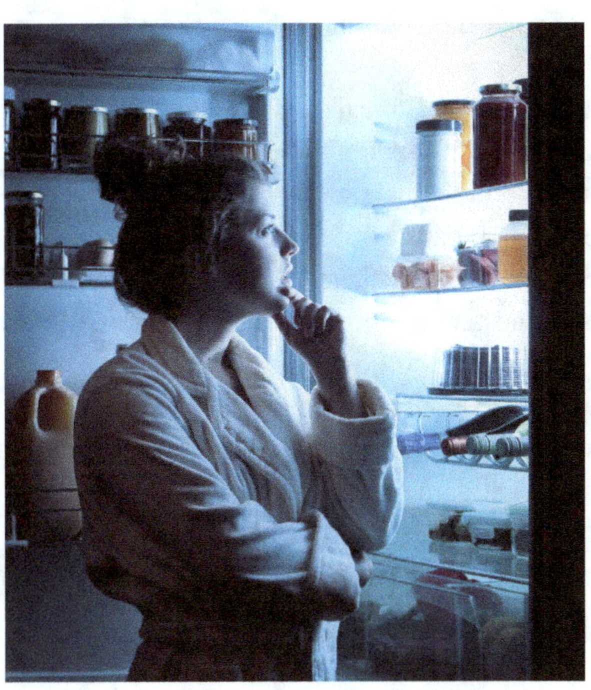

Which foods help with acid reflux during pregnancy?

Eating certain foods can help pregnant women manage acid reflux symptoms, and these options include

- Yogurt.
- Ginger tea.
- Almonds.
- Pineapple.
- Soups and smoothies that are easy to digest.

Four or five small meals a day is better for a pregnant woman with reflux than three large meals.

Bloating and constipation - Pregnant women often experience bloating and constipation. According to statistics, their prevalence ranges from 16 to 39% in each trimester of pregnancy and 6 to 12 weeks postpartum.

Bloating and constipation during pregnancy are also caused by hormonal changes that affect the motility of the small and large intestines.

Increased progesterone concentrations play a major role in reducing the activity of colon smooth muscle, but other hormones may also be involved.

Pregnant women also experience constipation for the same reasons as the general population.

In particular, a reduction in physical activity due to pregnancy complications and the prescription of iron supplements for iron deficiency may be recommended; both of these interventions can contribute to constipation.

What causes constipation during pregnancy?

Progesterone: A woman's body produces more of the hormone progesterone when she is pregnant.
Progesterone relaxes her intestines so that they don't work too hard to squeeze waste through her body. Slowing down gives your body more time to absorb nutrients and water from the food you eat.

The longer food stays in your intestines, the more time your colon has to absorb moisture from it. When a pregnant woman tries to go to the bathroom, the stool dries up and becomes difficult to pass.

Fetus: A growing fetus makes a woman's uterus heavier. This extra weight can put more pressure on her intestines, making it harder for waste to leave her body.

Iron from a prenatal vitamin: The iron a pregnant woman gets from a prenatal vitamin helps the body produce the blood needed to circulate oxygen throughout the expectant mother's body and her baby's body. However, too much iron can make it difficult for bacteria in the intestines to break down food.

Not having enough water to soften the waste that gets stuck in the woman's intestines only exacerbates the problem. Waste can build up and cause constipation.

Lifestyle: Diet, the amount of fluids she drinks each day, and the amount of exercise she does all play an important role in the onset of constipation.

Most pregnant people don't eat enough fiber, drink enough water, or exercise to help the digestive system eliminate toxins from the body.

How is constipation treated during pregnancy?

The first step in treating constipation is to increase the amount of fluids and fiber in your diet. Eating whole grains, fruits, and vegetables can often relieve constipation.

Good bathroom habits also help, especially the following

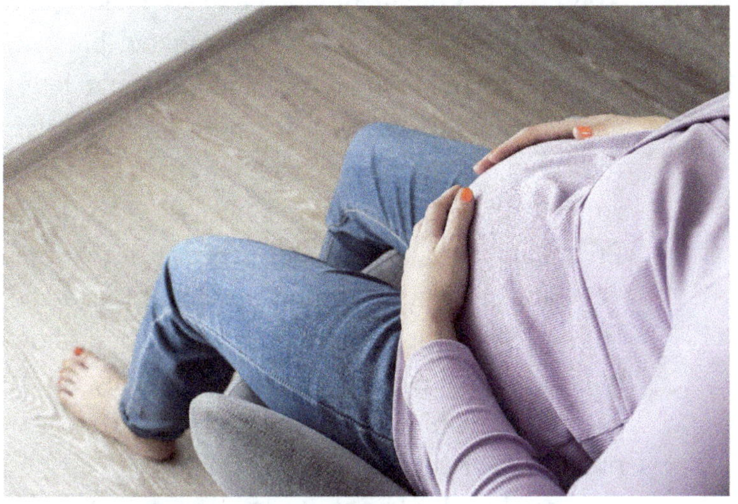

- Going to the bathroom as soon as you feel the urge - no need to wait and be patient.
- Eating and drinking, especially a hot drink at breakfast, can stimulate the urge to go.
- It is advisable to try to sit on the toilet about 20 minutes after eating, especially breakfast.
- Use a foot rest and sit on the toilet, leaning forward with your legs apart and your back straight.
- Avoid tension by consciously relaxing your abdominal muscles (think about making them "stick out").

How do you get rid of constipation during pregnancy?

- You can't tell pregnant women to stop taking the pregnancy hormones, it's not realistic, but you can help them make other changes that can help.
- You should eat 25 to 30 grams of fiber-rich foods every day: fiber can really help. Fiber softens the stool, making it easier to pass. Pregnant women can get fiber from fruits, vegetables, whole grains, beans, peas, and lentils. You should measure with them how many grams they get from the foods they eat. If pregnant women are constipated, they are probably not getting enough fiber.
- You need to drink eight to twelve cups of water a day: People say you need to drink eight cups of water a day. But eight cups is the minimum when a woman is pregnant. You need more fluids than usual to support the pregnancy and soften the stool. Water is best, but if a woman is not a fan, you can advise her to try other beverages. Skim milk, smoothies, tea, and juice with no added sugar are good options.
- Do moderate exercise for 20 to 30 minutes three times a week: sitting is not good for the bowels if a person is constipated. Of course, we do not mean heavy cardio training, but moderate physical activity, but it is desirable to have it.

- Try a different prenatal vitamin: The iron in the prenatal vitamin a pregnant woman takes may be too much for her digestive system.
- Remember that fiber is a type of nutrient that reduces the risk of disease and supports digestive health.
- There are several types of fiber found in different foods.
- Including a variety of fresh foods in your diet will ensure that you get enough fiber.

CHAPTER 7: HOW MUCH SHOULD A NEW MOTHER EAT?

Most new moms need between 1,800 and 2,200 calories a day for the first few months after giving birth.

And if they are underweight, exercise more than 45 minutes a day, or breastfeed more than one baby, this number may be higher.

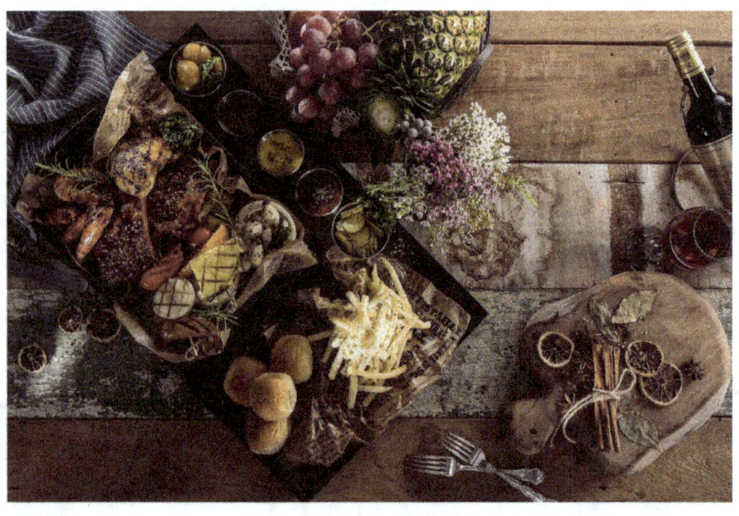

The estimated energy requirements (i.e. caloric intake) based on the mother's age, weight, height, and level of physical activity, and specifically for lactating women, are

- From 0 to 6 months postpartum - 330 kcal more than non-lactating women. This is based on the energy expenditure of exclusive breastfeeding of 500 kcal/day (based on an average milk production of 1.6pt (780 ml) per day with an average energy content of 67 kcal/0.2pt/100 ml).
- From 7 to 12 months postpartum, this is 400 kcal more than women who do not breastfeed.
- For women with a healthy body mass index and average height, this translates into a total energy requirement of 2,130 to 2,730 kcal/day during the first six months of lactation and 2,200 to 2,800 kcal/day thereafter, depending on the mother's age, weight, height, and activity level. A woman's energy needs also depend on the timing and rate of weaning.
- The recommended intake of protein during the first six months of lactation is the same as during pregnancy, 2.5 oz (71 g) per day. This amount is based on the volume of milk (approximately 1.6pt (780ml) per day) and the average protein content of milk 0.035oz/0.2pt (1g/100ml). But remember that the mother's diet does not affect the amount of protein in breast milk. Unlike fats, the amount of fat in a woman's diet has a minimal effect on the amount of fatty acids in breast milk. Foods such

as beans, seafood, lean meat, eggs, and soy products are rich in protein, which helps the body recover from childbirth.

- Fruits, vegetables, legumes, and whole grains (corn, millet, oats, wheat, and uncooked rice). At least 14oz/day (400g) (5 servings) of fruits and vegetables per day, excluding potatoes, cassava, and other starchy root vegetables.
- Eat fresh fruits and vegetables between meals.
- Fat should account for less than 30% of total energy intake.
- Favor unsaturated fats, such as those found in fish, avocados and nuts, and sunflower, soybean, canola and olive oils.
- Consume less than 0.18oz (5g) of salt per day (equivalent to one teaspoon).
- Free sugars should make up less than 10% of total energy intake, which is 1.8oz (50g) (or 12 teaspoons without the tip).

How should a woman eat if she wants to lose weight? How do you do this without interfering with proper recovery, especially if you are breastfeeding?

Most new mothers lose about 4lb (2kg) of weight per month.

Some may be tempted to go on a diet to speed up the process, but this is not a good idea. Explain to them that if they get less than 1,800 calories a day, their energy levels and mood will drop dramatically. So the best thing to do is to stick to a healthy, balanced eating plan and start exercising when their health allows.

You need to be careful with these products:

Alcohol: Experts have different opinions on how safe it is for your baby and how long you should wait to breastfeed after drinking alcohol.

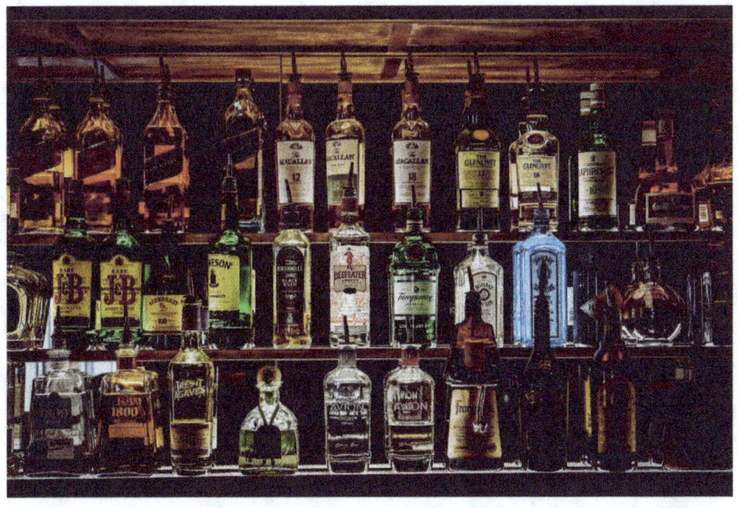

It is recommended that the baby should avoid contact with alcohol by waiting to feed for two hours after a single drink (0.75pt (355ml) of beer, or 0.3pt (148ml) of wine or 0.09pt (42ml) of liquor). If a woman drinks more than a single drink, she should generally refrain from breastfeeding for an additional two hours for each drink.

There is no need to express and discard milk after drinking alcohol, unless women experience an uncomfortable lump in the breast before enough time has passed for the alcohol to leave the body.

But even with this information, it is better not to recommend alcohol. Finally, alcohol consumption can impair the ability to feed and care for a child, so it should be avoided regardless of how the baby is fed.

Nicotine.

The baby's daily dose of nicotine is less than 5% of the mother's. This is the first number. Smoking 10 to 20 cigarettes a day is equivalent to about 0.5 mg of nicotine in 2 pints (1 liter) of milk, which is equivalent to a dose of 6 to 7.5 mg of nicotine in an adult. If consumed gradually throughout the day, the newborn will metabolize nicotine in the liver and excrete it through the kidneys.

Caffeine:

A nursing mother who drinks more than 3 cups (1.5pt (710 ml)) of coffee or soda a day may disrupt her baby's sleep and temperament (i.e., she may be irritable). However, some infants are sensitive to caffeine and become irritable or have trouble sleeping with even small amounts of caffeine. An infant's sensitivity to caffeine usually diminishes over time because newborns' excretion of caffeine is slow at first, but increases to adult levels by three to five months.

What remains unchanged is the avoidance of certain fish:
Swordfish, shark, king mackerel and tilefish, as these fish are high in mercury.
We recommend 226 to 340 grams per week of low-mercury fish and shellfish, including canned light tuna, salmon, pollock, catfish and shrimp.
You can also add one serving per week of bluefish, white tuna, and yellowfin tuna to your diet.

Vitamins - Fat-soluble and water-soluble vitamins are excreted in milk. Therefore, the need for most vitamins increases during lactation. Chronic dietary deficiency leads to depletion of maternal stores of some vitamins.
For women who eat a balanced diet, the increased nutrient requirements can be met by increasing the total food intake.
Some restrictive diets may require supplementation.

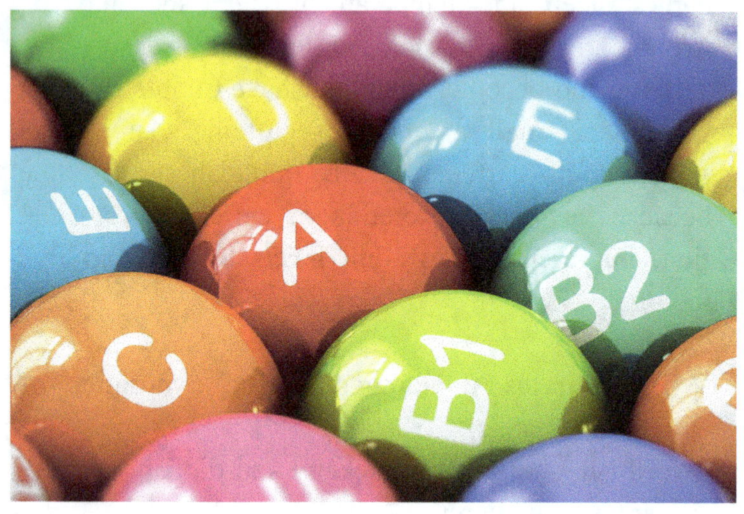

Weight Loss Diet - once lactation is established, overweight women can limit their energy intake to 500 kcal/day and perform aerobic exercise four days a week, if their condition allows, to promote weight loss of 1lb1.6oz (0.5kg) per week without compromising milk supply.

Rarely, the syndrome of "lactational ketoacidosis" has been reported in breastfeeding women, usually associated with restrictive diets and especially low carbohydrate intake. Symptoms and signs include nausea, vomiting, and abdominal pain.

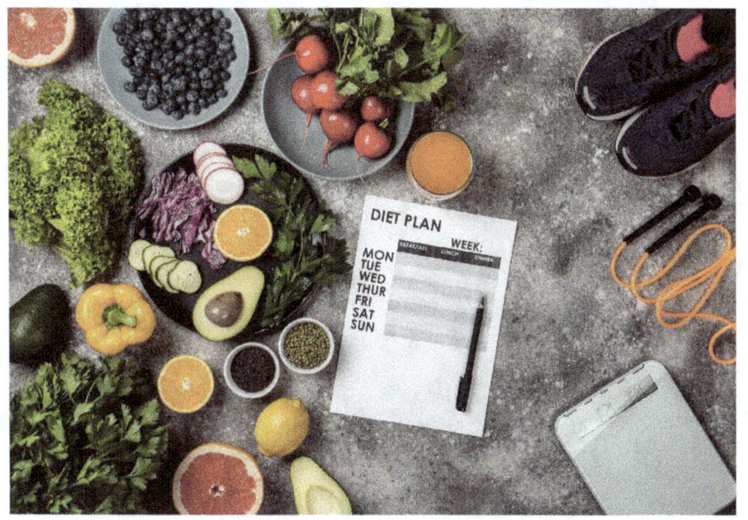

It is thought to be a form of fasting ketosis accelerated by the increased energy requirements of lactating women.

Vegetarian diet. Women who breastfeed and follow a vegetarian diet require different levels of dietary restrictions (e.g., ovo- or lacto-vegetarian) and may need to supplement with calcium, vitamin D, and vitamin B12 to ensure that they meet the recommended levels of these nutrients.

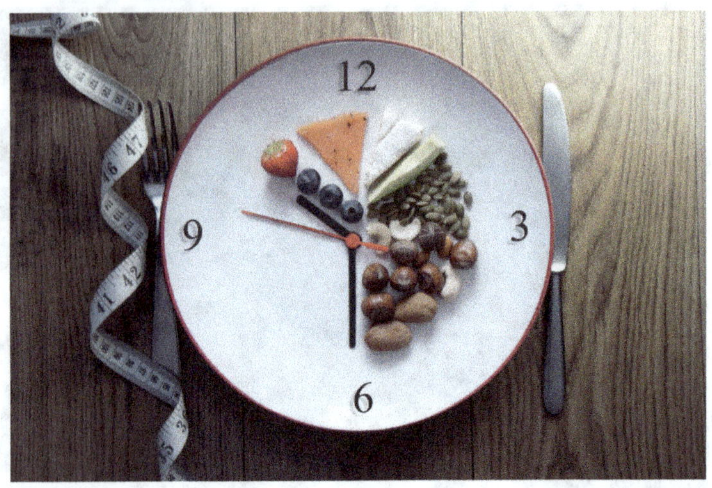

Vegan diet - healthy women who do not eat meat, chicken, fish, or dairy products should take vitamin supplements containing vitamin B12. Most commercially available multivitamins contain a sufficient dose of B12.

Fasting - Short-term fasting does not actually reduce milk production, but may have a slight effect on milk composition. Metabolic adaptations during short-term fasting preserve milk production, while prolonged fasting can negatively affect milk quality in lactating women. Thus, lactating women may be exempt from fasting during Ramadan for health reasons.

CHAPTER 8: THE IMPACT OF LACTATION

- First, there is a mild, gradual weight loss that usually occurs during the first 6 months after childbirth. Factors that contribute to postpartum weight loss include: weight gain during pregnancy, pre-pregnancy weight, age, race, smoking, exercise, and return to work.
- The second is muscle mass. The muscle mass of women who eat well is maintained during the first 6 months of breastfeeding.
- Third, hair loss after childbirth.

There are the following stages of hair growth:
- Anagen (i.e. the "growth" stage).
- Telogen (this is the "resting" stage).

Pregnancy slows down the transition from anagen to telogen.

In 1-5 months after childbirth, the percentage of telogenic hair increases and hair loss occurs (so-called telogenic alopecia), lasting up to 15 months.

A slight or moderate decrease in the energy intake of a lactating woman (at least 1500 kcal/day) has a limited effect on milk yield.

However, more severe malnutrition (less than 1500 kcal/day) can have a significant impact on milk production.

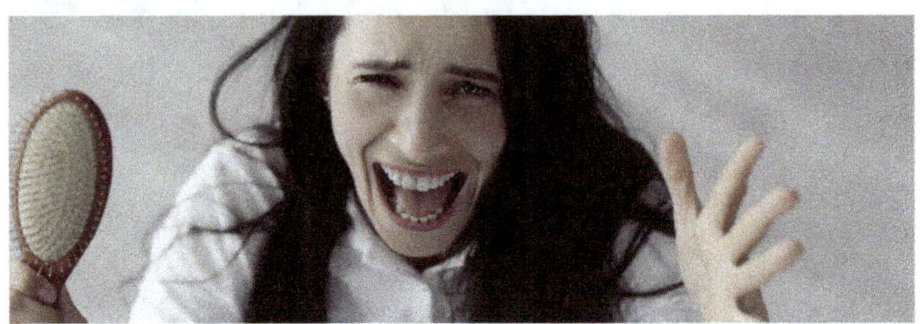

And in what situations can we talk about a lactating mother's diet?

The diet should be varied and include all healthy food groups. It should be remembered that a breastfeeding woman should eat 330 kcal/day more than a non-breastfeeding woman from birth to 6 months postpartum, and 400 kcal/day more than a non-breastfeeding woman from 7 to 12 months postpartum. There is no such thing as a "nursing mother's diet. A mother's diet does not prevent food allergies in her child.

However, there is a condition in children called **allergic proctocolitis** that is triggered by food proteins.

In this condition, a woman may indeed be advised to eliminate trigger foods such as cow's milk, eggs, soy, corn, as these are the most common triggers. But you don't have to eliminate everything all at once. It is enough to do it step by step and see if there is a result. Of course, if the clinical picture of proctocolitis in a child allows you to exclude foods step by step, because sometimes it has to be done all at once.

Breast milk is a living substance that changes its composition depending on: the time of day, the age of the child, and the child's need for food and fluids.

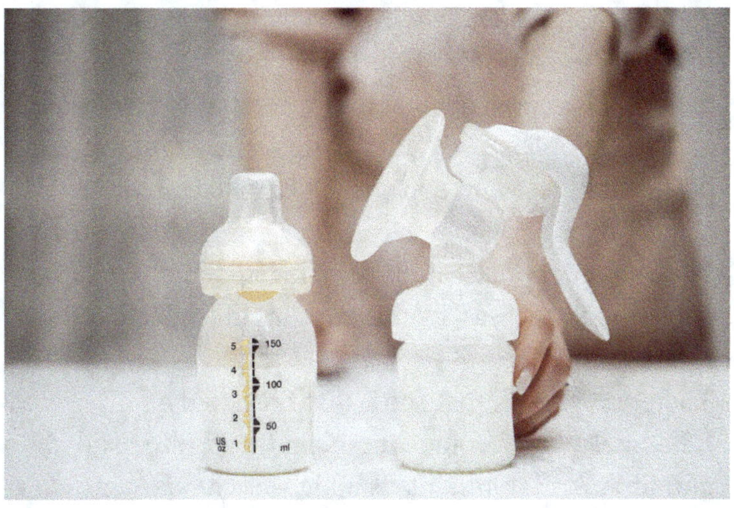

Milk produced in the morning is different from milk produced in the evening.

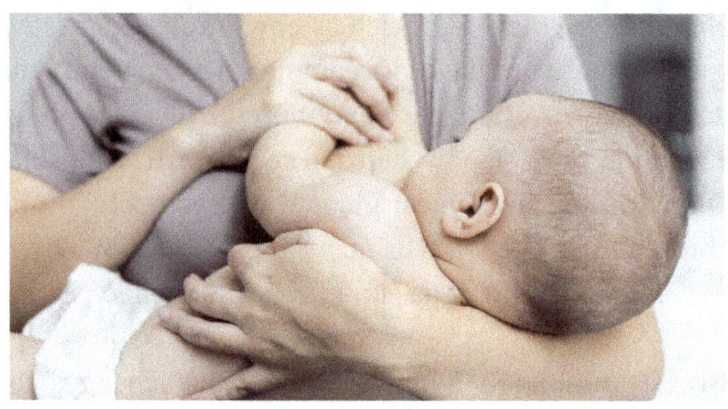

And in the process of feeding, it also changes its composition, for example, the amount of fat and calories in it gradually increases by the end of feeding, making the baby feel full. Breast milk contains more than 500 components that are beneficial for the health and development of the child, and a significant portion of these components CANNOT be reproduced chemically.

For example, breast milk contains appetite-regulating compounds such as leptin and ghrelin, which are not found in formula.

There are studies that show that breastfed children are less likely to become obese in the future, and the ghrelin in breast milk plays a big role in this.

The hormone melatonin, which is responsible for sleep, increases in evening milk. Daytime milk contains many amino acids that promote activity.

Iron in milk is highest at noon and vitamin E in the evening. Magnesium, zinc, potassium and sodium are highest in the morning. This means that the nutritional value is different at different times of the day.

Breast milk has been shown to have four functions:
- maturation,
- immunomodeling,
- anti-inflammatory,
- and antimicrobial.

Breastfeeding is not only about building immunity, but also about the emotional bond between mother and child.

It's also about convenience and economy, because you can breastfeed your child anytime, anywhere, and you don't have to buy formula, prepare it, wash bottles, etc.

The composition of breast milk is varied:
- **Proteins.** There are two groups: whey proteins - lactoferrin, secretory immunoglobulin A, lysozyme and alpha-lactalbumin, which is the main whey protein, and the second group - casein. The ratio of whey proteins to casein changes during lactation, initially it is 80/20, and after the age of 3 months it is 50/50.

- **Fats, also known as lipids**. They are characterized by a high content of palmitic and oleic acids. They are the most variable macronutrient in milk, but why?

  First, at the end of a feeding there is 2-3 times more fat than at the beginning of the feeding.

  Second, the composition of fats is much lower in night and morning feeds than in day and evening feeds. Third, the composition of fats depends on the amount of protein consumed by the mother.

  Finally, the fatty acid profile varies depending on the mother's diet, especially in the case of long-chain polyunsaturated fatty acids.

- The main **carbohydrate** in breast milk is B-lactose, and its concentration is the least variable of the macronutrients.

  Its composition depends on the amount of milk and the stage of lactation. That is, the more milk, the more lactose. And as for the stage of lactation, colostrum contains the least lactose and gradually increases until the 4th month of lactation.

  In addition to lactose, there are also carbohydrates - oligosaccharides, they are non-caloric biologically active factors, their composition also depends on the stage of lactation, most of them are in colostrum, and their amount gradually decreases by 20% by the thirtieth day from the beginning of lactation. There are also small amounts of glucose and galactose in breast milk. What is their role in all this?

Lactose satisfies 40% of the baby's energy needs, it is necessary for the absorption of calcium, magnesium, zinc, iron, but its most important role is in the development of the central nervous system. What is the role of oligosaccharides?

They contain a "bifidus factor" for the growth of bifidus bacteria, which in turn produce lactic acid to suppress the growth of pathogens in the intestinal, respiratory and urinary tracts.

- **Biologically active components** of breast milk include hormones, enzymes, immune complexes, and numerous regulatory factors.

  They help newborns overcome birth stress faster and adapt better to new living conditions. These substances contribute to normal digestion, proper metabolism, initial immune support and the formation of a child's protective intestinal bifidus microflora, and later - a full-fledged immune system.

- **Vitamins and macronutrients.**

DAILY NUTRITIONAL REQUIREMENTS DURING LACTATION (for ages over 19)

- Calorie estimates - 2200-2400 kcal
- Protein - 71 g (10 to 30% kcal)
- Carbohydrates - 210 g (45 to 65% kcal)
- Fiber - 31-34 g (14 g/1000 kcal)
- Added sugars - <10% kcal
- Total lipid - 25-35% kcal
- Saturated fats - <10% kcal
- Linolenic acid - 1.3 g
- Linoleic acid - 13 g
- Calcium - 1000 mg
- Iron - 9 mg
- Magnesium - 310-320 mg
- Phosphorus - 700 mg
- Potassium - 2800 mg
- Sodium - 2300 mg
- Zinc - 12 mg
- Iodine - 290 mcg
- Selenium [1] - 70 mcg
- Vitamin A - 1300 mcg
- Vitamin D - 15 mcg (600 international units)
- Vitamin E (as AT) - 19 mg
- Vitamin K - 90 mcg
- Vitamin C - 120 mg
- Thiamine - 1.4 mg
- Riboflavin - 1.6 mg
- Niacin - 17 mg

- Vitamin B6 - 2 mg
- Vitamin B12 - 2.8 mcg
- Choline - 550 mg
- Folic acid - 500 mcg

CLOSING REMARKS

Dear mom-to-be,
Congratulations on your journey through nutrition during pregnancy and breastfeeding! We've learned a lot together, discovered new ways to eat well, and found a source of inspiration.

Now that you've finished this book, I hope you feel more confident and know how to help you and your baby be healthy and strong. Eating is not only for your body, but also for your baby.

Every bite and sip you give your baby becomes part of their growth and development. This connects us to ancient traditions when nutrition was the source of life and health.

Good nutrition is not a restriction; it's an opportunity to feel strong, energized, and full of life. It's an investment in your baby's future.

May every day of your motherhood be joyful and well-being. May these moments of nourishment be a time of physical and mental bonding with your baby.

I would really appreciate it if you could **share your impression of the program in an amazon review**.

Your experience can inspire others and motivate long-term changes in their eating habits.

Proud of you,
your Valerie Spark